SUSAN O'BRIEN is an author, baker, gourmet cook, food management consultant, cooking instructor, product development consultant, guest speaker, and the owner of two businesses, O'Brien's Kitchen and O'Brien's Consulting, LLC. She lives in Gig Harbor, Washington.

The
GLUTEN-FREE
VEGAN

The
GLUTEN-FREE
VEGAN

150

Delicious Gluten-Free,
Animal-Free Recipes

SUSAN O'BRIEN

Da Capo
LIFE
LONG

A MEMBER OF THE PERSEUS BOOKS GROUP

Copyright © 2007 by Susan O'Brien

Designed by Pauline Neuwirth, Neuwirth & Associates, Inc.
Set in 11 point Baskerville MT by the Perseus Books Group

Cataloging-in-Publication data for this book is available from the Library of Congress.

ISBN: 978-1-60094-032-3

Published by Da Capo Press
A Member of the Perseus Books Group
www.dacapopress.com

Note: The information in this book is true and complete to the best of our knowledge.
This book is intended only as an informative guide for those wishing to know more
about health issues. In no way is this book intended to replace, countermand, or conflict
with the advice given to you by your own physician. The ultimate decision concerning
care should be made between you and your doctor. We strongly recommend you follow
his or her advice. Information in this book is general and is offered with no guarantees
on the part of the authors or Da Capo Press. The authors and publisher disclaim all
liability in connection with the use of this book. The names and identifying details
of people associated with events described in this book have been changed. Any
similarity to actual persons is coincidental.

Da Capo Press books are available at special discounts for bulk purchases in
the U.S. by corporations, institutions, and other organizations. For more
information, please contact the Special Markets Department at the Perseus
Books Group, 2300 Chestnut Street, Suite 200, Philadelphia, PA, 19103, or
call (800) 2810-4145, ext. 5000, or e-mail special.markets@perseusbooks.com.

10 9 8 7 6 5

This book is dedicated to
my loving community of friends and family
with gratitude

CONTENTS

Preface by Barb Schiltz, RN, MS, CN   xi
Introduction   xiii

Eating Gluten-Free, Vegan, . . . and Healthy   1
   Why Vegan?   1
   Organic Foods   1
   GMO Foods   2
   Raw Foods   2
   Dairy Alternatives and Casein   3
   Gluten-Free, Casein-Free Diet for Autism Spectrum Disorders   4
   Celiac Disease   4
   The Oat Debate   5
   The Glycemic Index   5
   Sugar Alternatives   6
   Shortenings   8
   Oils   8
   Soy, Rice, Coconut, and Almond Milk   8
   Coconut Milk   9
   Egg Substitutes   9
   Gluten / Wheat Substitutes   10
   Foods to Avoid if on a Gluten-Free Diet   13
   Other Ingredients   13
   Cooking Guide for Grains   15

THE RECIPES   17

Appetizers   19
Soups   29

Salads   41
Vegetable and Side Dishes   55
Main Dishes   83
Breakfast Foods   109
Breads, Muffins, Scones, and Crusts   119
Desserts   133
Beverages   157
Sauces and Condiments   167

Resources
    Where Can You Find Common Ingredients Used in This Book?   179
    Resource Guide for Gluten-Free, Vegan Products   181

Acknowledgments   183
Index   185

PREFACE

How can you be a healthy vegan and also be gluten free? This can be a daunting task! Most vegans eat quite a lot of wheat and other gluten whole grains for their healthy carbohydrate content, along with some protein, too. In the past five years, I have seen many patients who have been put on a gluten-free diet for health reasons. Joint pain and digestive complaints are common symptoms of people who are gluten sensitive. Even those who have minor symptoms are surprised to find that, when they avoid gluten for several weeks, they feel better than they ever thought they could feel!

It is common for me to meet people everywhere (not just in my nutrition practice) who are struggling to find grains that are both satisfying and tasty. LOOK NO FURTHER! *The Gluten-Free Vegan* is your answer. Sue has made this an easy and delicious task. You no longer have to restrict your grains to rice and corn! Just try a new recipe every week and, before you know it, being a gluten-free vegan will be no big deal.

Sue uses grains that are new to most people. For example, quinoa (pronounced "keen-wa") is a South American food that has a higher protein content than most grains. It is technically not a grain but looks and tastes like a grain and so is treated as one. And sorghum flour is a great substitute for wheat when baking. I was impressed when I tried it for the first time last year when Sue's cookbook *Gluten-Free, Sugar-Free Cooking* [third edition] was published. My gluten-free patients were thrilled to find this cookbook.

Even if you are not a vegan, you should try these recipes. Perhaps you or other family members have some food allergies . . . or, maybe you would like to have one or two vegetarian meals each week, just for health reasons. Then this is the cookbook for you. *The Gluten-Free Vegan* will help you to prepare wonderful recipes for you and your family. I plan to recommend this cookbook to my patients with food allergies or gluten sensitivities, and also to those who desire to prepare and eat more healthy meals. It will finally be easier when I suggest that my vegan patients try to avoid gluten for a trial period: a copy of Sue's book will be the first thing they purchase!

Bon appétit,

BARB SCHILTZ, RN, MS, CN

INTRODUCTION

THIS IS MY fourth cookbook. All have been gluten free, but this is my first vegan cookbook. Writing this book has been a wonderful experience for me, in that it has allowed me the opportunity to be a pioneer as a cook. Writing a vegan cookbook is no easy feat, but writing a *gluten-free, vegan* cookbook has truly been a creative experience. It has allowed me to "think outside the box" and to engage my community in the process of testing all of these recipes.

I have been amazed at how well I feel as a result of eating the recipes created for this book. I am not saying by any means that if you prepare and consume the recipes in this book that you have found a "magic potion" that will cure your ills, but I can tell you that my energy level is sustained throughout the day, and that my body doesn't have to work so hard to perform elimination functions because I am eating so many fruits and vegetables as well as healthy fats and legumes. I also feel great because I am gluten free, dairy free and do not feel deprived in any way. In fact, I feel grateful— grateful that I am well and able to enjoy eating foods that support my well-being. I have a family history of high cholesterol, and the only change I made over the past year was to eat the foods I developed for this cookbook. My latest cholesterol work-up shows my total cholesterol is just over 200 mg/dL, but my HDL is at an all-time high of 99 mg/dL. The American Heart Association recommends total cholesterol under 200 mg/dL and an HDL 40mg/dL or higher.

This work represents what I am most passionate about. The difficult part of this experience was finding the balance between writing this book, my personal life, and my other full-time job. I worked all day and then headed straight to the kitchen each night to develop new recipes to share with you. That part of this experience was wonderful, creating recipes that I hope will excite you, draw you into the kitchen, and provide you with new ideas on how to eat well while gluten free. But it was also exhausting, as I wanted the very best I could offer, and it took a tremendous amount of effort. Overall, writing this book has been a gift to me and, I hope, to you as well.

I know how challenging it can be to eliminate gluten from your diet. I also know how fantastic it can be to finally feel well, to wake up without the "foggy brain" or to be able to remember something as simple as a name. If you are gluten intolerant or have a gluten allergy, perhaps you have experienced some of these symptoms: constipation, diarrhea, bloating, or abdominal cramping. You may have experienced other symptoms, too, perhaps migraine headaches, body aches, fibromyalgia, or chronic fatigue. So many of the medical concerns we face today are not from stress or lifestyle (although that can be the case); many of the symptoms I mentioned above are a consequence of diet, of our eating foods that our body cannot tolerate. Have you heard or read about gluten intolerance? Celiac disease? Gluten sensitivity? Crohn's disease? There are several medical conditions that are directly linked to gluten intolerance/allergies, yet many people go undiagnosed or misdiagnosed, and thus they suffer needlessly because they don't know that what they are eating is keeping them from being healthy. Read the papers, listen to the news, search the Internet with the keyword "gluten"—you will see what I mean. Ten out of every one hundred people have some sort of problem with gluten. That's a huge number of people in this country alone. Are you one of those people? But, suspecting or knowing that gluten is the culprit, do you wonder what you *can* eat? Do you walk around your kitchen opening up cupboards or stand in front of your refrigerator with the door open, just looking inside? I have been there. I was frustrated, hungry, upset that I couldn't eat my favorite foods, and not sure what in the heck I could eat.

That was eight years ago. Today I no longer crave foods that contain gluten. I know how to eat to support my health and to cook foods that taste delicious. I know what to make when I need a quick pick-me-up, in a hurry, and what to make when I really want to "go the extra mile" to make something special. I now include more raw, fresh foods in my diet, making raw soups, pies, smoothies, and more. I now eat more fruits and vegetables than I ate in my entire childhood, and they are not canned or processed, or overcooked, stripping them of their nutrients. They are organic, and prepared with loving energy that gives back the energy to me so that I can maintain my wellness.

I cook with herbs and spices and eat healthy nuts and blueberries and other foods that not only sustain my health but protect me from cancer, heart disease, strokes, autoimmune disorders, and more. Being a vegan doesn't mean all you eat is brown rice and baked potatoes (I once heard someone say those two foods are the most common foods vegans eat). The recipes in this book are chock full of flavors and textures and snap, crackle, and crunch! Perhaps in my past I relied too heavily on one ingredient to provide the main flavor of the dish, whereas now I use many different herbs and spices and mix flavors that I never considered before. For example, today I combine bananas and applesauce to replace eggs in a recipe that also may contain organic cocoa or vegan chocolate chips. This combination may sound funny, but I encourage you to try the brownies found on page 138. I think you will find this combination quite delicious!

So, take off. Roll up your sleeves, and dig in. I challenge you to be creative in your kitchen, and to do so with a sense of humor and an open mind. The recipes I have created are only a starting point. They have all been tried out by loving friends, family members, colleagues, strangers, and those in the community who support my efforts. I hope you will feel free to experiment with these recipes so that they support YOUR wellness. I believe the loving energy we infuse into the food we prepare and eat is what helps us live a healthy life. I hope you take the time to prepare your food with love, and share it with your friends, family, and community so they, too, can feel the energy of life.

Be well,

Susan O'Brien
May 2007

The
GLUTEN-FREE
VEGAN

EATING GLUTEN-FREE, VEGAN, . . . AND HEALTHY

WHY VEGAN?

To BE VEGAN means that you eat only those foods that are absolutely animal free: no meat, eggs, dairy products, or animal-derived ingredients such as gelatin.

People choose to become vegans for several reasons—health and wellness, environmental concerns, political reasons, or ethical decisions. Many people with medical problems have turned to a vegan diet. Today, more than ever, there is evidence that America's rising obesity is due to the overconsumption of saturated fats and high-cholesterol foods. New York State has banned trans fats from restaurants, and snack food manufacturers are scrambling to come up with non-trans-fat processed products that will appeal to the mass market.

What's wrong with fruits, vegetables, nuts, and other plant foods, I ask? You don't have to sacrifice your health to enjoy good foods.

So, health and wellness are two reasons that people become vegans. In this book I am not going to go into the other reasons, as my focus is to bring you healthy, delicious recipes that will support your health and wellness, and delight your senses.

ORGANIC FOODS

I HIGHLY RECOMMEND that you choose organic foods whenever possible. I know that, in some places around the country, this is a difficult proposition, but I am happy to report that more and more mainstream stores are stocking organic produce and other grocery items. This is great. However, whenever you can, I recommend that you buy from your local organic farms. To do so, not only supports the farms, it also ensures the foods you purchase are at their freshest. I strongly recommend you buy the following fruits and veggies organic, for they are the produce most contaminated with pesticides:

- ▶ Apples
- ▶ Celery
- ▶ Cherries
- ▶ Grapes
- ▶ Lettuce
- ▶ Nectarines

- ▶ Pears
- ▶ Potatoes
- ▶ Spinach
- ▶ Strawberries
- ▶ Bell Peppers

I don't state in every recipe that the veggies or fruits need to be organic, but that's what I use, and I hope you will, too.

When buying organic, be sure the label says "100 percent organic." Some food labels state they are "organic" but these may contain 5 percent of nonorganic substances. Only "100 percent organic" guarantees that all the ingredients are organic.

If you want to save money, the following conventionally produced fruits and veggies are the least contaminated:

- ▶ Asparagus
- ▶ Avocados
- ▶ Bananas
- ▶ Cabbage
- ▶ Kiwis

- ▶ Mangoes
- ▶ Onions
- ▶ Papayas
- ▶ Peas
- ▶ Pineapples

For a more complete list of fruits and vegetables that it is important to buy organic and strategies for buying organic and locally-grown foods, check out Cindy Burke's *To Buy or Not to Buy Organic*.

GMO FOODS

GMO is short for "genetically engineered and modified organisms." I do not intentionally use any foods in my cookbook, or in my home, that are GMO. These foods are a threat to all of us, in my opinion, and also pose a threat to our environment and our agricultural heritage. I encourage you to avoid these foods, and to read labels—look for "GMO free."

RAW FOODS

THERE IS CURRENTLY a movement toward consuming raw foods. I don't believe this is a passing fad or a craze. I think many people have made a decision to eat all or some of their food raw because, in that form, the nutrients remain intact. Heating foods kills healthy bacteria and lowers the nutritional value. I have included several raw food recipes in this book. I hope you will give them a try. The Tropical Pudding Pie is a wonderful dessert I am sure you will enjoy.

DAIRY ALTERNATIVES AND CASEIN

FOR VEGANS, DAIRY is not an option, as it comes from animals. People who are not vegan may wish to eat a more healthful diet or may need to be casein/caseinate free. Many people need to avoid lactose. Here is a list of foods that do contain casein and/or lactose, and a list of alternatives.

■ Foods to Avoid if on a Vegan, Dairy-Free, or Casein-Free Diet

Read the labels for these items very carefully, and make sure they are specifically "vegan," as even if they appear to be dairy-free (yes, even if labeled "pareve"), they may contain casein.

- ▶ Cow's milk, cream, and half-and-half
- ▶ Cheese, including soy or rice cheese (many of which contain casein)
- ▶ Yogurt
- ▶ Butter and some margarines
- ▶ Ice cream, ice milk, sherbet, and frozen yogurt
- ▶ Whipped toppings
- ▶ Pudding, custard, and other creamy desserts
- ▶ Creamed soups, vegetables, sauces, and gravies, as well as the uncreamed kind
- ▶ Baking and eating chocolate (check label for whether they were made on machinery that processes milk products, which can leave behind traces of milk)
- ▶ All sheep's and goat's milks, and products made from those milks
- ▶ Bottled dressings, including mayonnaise-like dressings
- ▶ Pasta sauces
- ▶ Over-the-counter vitamins and other capsules/pills (may contain lactose as a nonactive ingredient)

■ Alternatives

- ▶ Rice milk, soy milk, coconut milk, nut milks, and hemp milk
- ▶ Soy yogurt
- ▶ Tofutti brand products, including Tofutti sour cream, cream cheese, frozen confections, etc.

- ► Coconut oil and maple butter
- ► Rice Dream frozen confections (double-check labels for casein)
- ► Other brands of soy frozen confections (check labels)
- ► Italian water ices (check the label to be certain they are dairy-free)
- ► Sorbet (again, check the label)
- ► Tropical Source brand chocolate and chocolate chips
- ► Earth Balance Buttery Spread/Shortening and Spectrum Shortening
- ► *Specifically vegan* baked goods, snacks, cereals, sauces, dressings, soups, and other packaged foods
- ► Enjoy Life Foods semi-sweet chocolate chips

GLUTEN-FREE, CASEIN-FREE DIET FOR AUTISM SPECTRUM DISORDERS

SEVERAL STUDIES HAVE been conducted regarding the benefits of a gluten-free, casein-free (gf/cf) diet for people diagnosed with autism spectrum conditions. The following Web sites may be of interest to you if you are looking for more information on the benefits of a gluten-free, casein-free diet for these conditions:

- ► ANDI (Autism Network for Dietary Intervention)—www.autismNDI.com
- ► The GFCF Diet Support Group—www.gfcfdiet.com
- ► The NIH Web site on Autism Spectrum Disorders— www.nimh.nih.gov/public/autism.cfm
- ► The Center for the Study of Autism—www.AutismResearchInstitute.com

CELIAC DISEASE

CELIAC DISEASE, OR sprue, is an autoimmune disease that affects the intestines. People who have celiac disease are not able to break down the proteins in gluten, which is found in wheat, rye, and barley. Since wheat is a staple in the United States, it is in virtually everything, from pasta, breads, and cereals to sauces and soups to desserts. For those who have celiac disease, this can have devastating effects. Depending on the severity of the condition, a person with celiac sprue may have mild or life-threatening reactions to eating foods that contain gluten.

USA Today ran a full-page story in November 2006 regarding the prevalence of celiac disease, and how frequently it is misdiagnosed. A study conducted in 2004 estimates that as many as 1 in 133 people in the United States may have celiac disease and are not aware of it. Some individuals have symptoms while others do not, but even without symptoms, damage may be going on inside that will manifest at some point later in life.

Several tests are available to determine if you have celiac disease, or an allergy or intolerance to gluten. Check with your doctor if you suspect you have one of these conditions, as there are diagnostic tests available. Once you know, you can make lifestyle changes that support your health, today and into the future.

When I first started on a gluten-free diet seven years ago, not many "safe" grain substitutes were available that tasted good and were good for me. Today, gluten-free foods are available all over the country—in restaurants, on airplanes, in grocery stores, and for sale through the Internet. The days of feeling deprived are over, and the time has come to celebrate a healthier way of eating!

THE OAT DEBATE

FOR MANY YEARS, oats have been off limits to celiacs and others with a gluten intolerance or allergy. The reason is based not on the oats themselves—they have been shown to be free of gluten—but on how they are processed: they experience cross-contamination with other products that contain gluten. Now that this is understood, some manufacturers have dedicated their equipment to the gluten-free production of oats. So, today there are new options for folks who wish to consume this valuable grain. Oats contain soluble-rich fiber that boosts energy, and aids in reducing cholesterol. There are several different kinds of oats, but if you want to be sure they are gluten-free, you need to buy them from a certified gluten-free manufacturer. Here are two that I have found to be very reliable:

www.glutenfreeoats.com
www.giftsofnature.net

THE GLYCEMIC INDEX

THE GLYCEMIC INDEX is a way of measuring the carbohydrate content of a food and how quickly it will raise your blood glucose (blood sugar) levels. All foods have a number on a scale of 0 to 100 that indicates their glycemic level. Those foods with highest numbers cause the greatest rise in blood sugar, and those with lower numbers, a smaller rise in blood sugar levels. A high GI value is 70 or more, a moderate GI value is 56-69, and a low GI value is 55 or less.

Foods high in carbohydrates, such as white flour, white potatoes, white rice, and treats made with refined sugars, are very high on the glycemic index. They digest very quickly in the intestine and cause a rapid increase in blood sugar. Other foods, such as apples, grapefruit, or pears are low on the glycemic scale and do not cause a rapid response of insulin from the pancreas. If you are trying to eat a healthy diet, it is good to consume foods that are lower on the glycemic index scale, to keep your blood sugars balanced.

Many sites on the Internet, such as www.glycemicindex.com, offer information about the glycemic index, as well as the index scale itself. If you are concerned with the amount of carbohydrates you are consuming, and wish to lower your intake of high glycemic carbs, look to the Internet for more information. There are also books available on this topic, such as *The New Glucose Revolution: The Authoritative Guide to the Glycemic Index* by Jennie Brand-Miller, PhD and Thomas M. S. Wolever, MD, PhD, and *The Good Carb Cookbook: Secrets of Eating Low on the Glycemic Index* by Sandra L. Woodruff.

SUGAR ALTERNATIVES

STAYING WITH THE health and wellness attitude, I have made 95 percent of the recipes in this book using a wonderful organic sweetener called agave nectar. It comes from the cactus plant, is very easily digested, and, due to its low rating on the glycemic index scale, is suitable for diabetics. It's rated 11 on the scale, and that is wonderful news, because it tastes fantastic, stores well in the cupboard, and can be easily substituted for refined sugar or even maple syrup. Other sweeteners include maple syrup, stevia, raw organic sugar, Sucanat, blackstrap molasses, brown rice syrup, and turbinado sugar. I personally use agave nectar in most of my recipes but occasionally will use brown rice syrup, molasses, maple syrup, or raw or organic sugar.

I have also used a fruit sweetener that is not available everywhere; if you choose to use it in your baking, check with your local health food store or perhaps Whole Foods, Fresh Fields, or Wild Oats. There are two brand names for the sweetener, which I have used with great success; they are Mystic Lake Dairy and Wax Orchards. Both products are made from all natural ingredients, a combination of peach, pear, and pineapple puree. This type of sweetener is higher on the glycemic index scale, so it has more of an effect on blood sugars than does the agave nectar. If you choose to use a fruit sweetener, you will have to cut the amount by ¼ cup, as it is much more concentrated than agave nectar.

When you use a sugar substitute, do so knowing which is best for you and your family. Here are some descriptions of them:

■ Brown Rice Syrup

The brand of brown rice syrup that is most readily available in grocery stores is Lundburg Farms. This family-owned farm has been making brown rice syrup for years and also has the best variety of rice and rice products, anywhere. I love their rice, especially their "brown rice," which is actually red in color. Brown rice syrup comes from rice, so it is safe for gluten-free vegans, and also contains water and fungal enzymes. I use this sweetener when I am making granola bars or brown rice pudding or need just a splash in a cup of tea. It is very sweet, so a little bit goes a long way.

■ Agave Cactus Nectar

As I mentioned, this is my sugar substitute of choice. I really love this sweetener! It comes from the pineapple-shaped core of the agave cactus, which is the same plant that is used to make tequila! There is no alcohol in agave nectar, but it has a very smooth, gentle sweetness that never leaves an aftertaste. This plant is native to Mexico and comes in three varieties: organic light, organic raw, and organic raw dark. The dark version contains more minerals, calcium, iron, potassium, and magnesium. The lighter version is filtered and has a lighter taste. One teaspoon of the cactus nectar contains 16 calories, 0 grams of fat, 5 grams of carbohydrates, 5 grams of sugar, 5 grams of sodium, and 0 grams of protein. To purchase agave nectar in bulk, see the reference list.

■ Maple Butter

This is amazing stuff. I just found out about it recently, so it's not used in a lot of the recipes in this book, but I highly recommend you pick some up and try it. I used it in the fudge recipe and a few others. It is made from pure maple syrup and invert maple syrup, which comes from the darker grade of maple syrup. Maple syrup comes in many forms; this is by far my favorite! Shady Maple Farms makes a certified organic maple butter that I love. They are in Canada, but I am sure you can find this product at your health food store. If they don't have it, ask them to get it for you. It's worth the wait. It's not cheap, but it is so condensed that you don't need much.

■ Molasses and Maple Syrup

In my previous cookbooks, I talked about honey in this section. Honey is not used in this cookbook because it is derived from bees and is therefore not vegan. I do recommend, though, that you substitute maple syrup in some of the recipes, if you are feeling creative; it has about the same consistency as the agave nectar and so can be used easily in place of agave. When using such liquids as molasses, maple syrup, and agave in a baking recipe, it is best to first mix the liquid ingredients (at room temperature) with the oil or nondairy margarine. I recommend beating these together until they become thick. This is important, as it will allow the oil and liquid to congeal before adding other ingredients to the mixture.

I rarely use molasses or maple syrup in my recipes, primarily because they are higher in sugar content, tend to raise blood sugar more rapidly, and I actually prefer the sweet taste of agave.

SHORTENINGS

■ Margarine, Organic Palm Shortening, and Coconut Oil

THERE ARE GOOD replacements for butter on the market these days. I use vegan margarine for best results in cookies, organic palm shortening in piecrusts, and coconut oil in other baking recipes. The Earth Balance brand of margarine and shortening is vegan, non-GMO, trans fat–free, dairy-free, and gluten-free. Look for both varieties in the dairy case at a health food store or in the natural foods fridge in a supermarket. Earth Balance Natural Buttery Spread works great for cookies, muffins, anything that you would use in place of butter. Earth Balance Natural Shortening is another option if you do not have any problems with soy. If you have an allergy to soy, you will want to consider using Spectrum Organic Shortening, which comes in a 24-ounce tub and is made from 100% organic, expeller-pressed palm oil. It can be found in the baking or oils section (doesn't need refrigeration) of health food stores and in supermarkets that carry natural products. This shortening, too, is vegan, dairy-free and gluten-free, has no cholesterol, and works wonderfully for piecrusts. Spectrum also carries organic coconut oil, sold off the shelf in a mayonnaise-like jar. They also make an organic margarine that's great for baking cookies and cakes. When choosing a vegan butter substitute, read your labels carefully, as you want to keep away from hydrogenated oils.

OILS

THERE ARE SEVERAL oils that I would recommend, but my two favorites are olive oil and grapeseed oil. Grapeseed oil contains vitamin C, vitamin E and beta-carotene, and carotin. It is reputed to contain antioxidants and to lower cholesterol. Studies have shown that it helps to raise the good cholesterol (HDL), and lower the bad cholesterol (LDL). One other benefit of grapeseed oil is that it can be used at high heat, so it is great for stir-fries and sautéing. Because this oil has a very light flavor, I also use it for baking. I use a tremendous amount of olive oil in this cookbook, as I love the flavor, the health benefits, and the fact that I can buy organic cold-pressed oil at my local grocery store. If you want to use grapeseed oil in place of olive oil, go ahead. I encourage you to be creative in your cooking. It's what makes it fun and keeps it interesting.

SOY, RICE, COCONUT, AND ALMOND MILK

I USE SOY milk in many of my recipes. It is low in fat and high in protein. I always buy the "unsweetened" versions, as the regular or flavored milks have a very high sugar content. Almond milk is sweet and can be used to replace cow's milk in recipes, too. I like rice milk on cereal for breakfast.

Hemp, rice milk, and soy milk can be used as a milk substitute in just about everything but foods that need to thicken, such as puddings and puddinglike pie fillings (you would need to add arrowroot powder, tapioca starch, or other natural gluten-free starch for the dish to thicken properly). I would recommend hemp, soy or rice milk as a thickener for gravies, but almond milk is delicious as a base for brown rice pudding. Be sure you refrigerate all of these milks after opening, and check the expiration date.

COCONUT MILK

I HAVE ADDED coconut milk to many of the recipes in this book and, even though I have not always indicated to use light coconut milk, that is my choice. The light version has less fat, and it works just as well as regular coconut milk—the flavor is not compromised at all. Years ago, we were told that coconut milk was bad for us because it contained too much fat. Research is now telling us the difference between this fat and others is that coconut milk is plant based, not animal based, and it contains lauric acid, which is very good for us. Literature has shown that it can aid weight loss, and promotes a healthy heart. Lauric acid is a fatty acid whose function is to form monolaurian. Monolaurian's properties are antibacterial, antiviral, and antimicrobial. Coconut oil has the largest concentration of lauric acid, but coconut milk also contains this acid, as does mother's milk. Its health benefits are vast, and I suggest you try substituting it for other milks in your own recipes.

Coconut water has recently made a splash on the market and it is reported to have many health benefits as well.

EGG SUBSTITUTES

MANY VEGAN EGG substitutes are available for use in your baked goods. I like Ener-G Foods egg replacer, which is made of potato starch, tapioca starch, and calcium carbonate/calcium lactate (which does not contain dairy lactose). To use Ener-G for one egg in a recipe, whisk together 1½ teaspoons of Ener-G with 2 tablespoons warm water, then add to the other liquid ingredients in the recipe. Double if the recipe calls for two eggs. Sometimes I don't like the results I get when I use this to replace two eggs, so instead, I will use Ener-G for one egg, and ¼ cup of applesauce for the other one.

You can also use the following to replace one egg:
▶ ¼ cup of applesauce
▶ 1 tablespoon of ground flaxseed beaten well with 3 tablespoons of water
▶ ½–1 ripe banana, mashed well

Another egg substitute is to mix ¼ cup of oil with ⅓ pound of silken tofu. This quantity equals 2 eggs and must be blended together well before incorporating into the rest of the ingredients.

GLUTEN/WHEAT SUBSTITUTES

As I MENTIONED previously, celiac disease, gluten intolerance, or allergies are all reasons why people are choosing other grains/flours than wheat, rye, or barley in the foods they consume. This book relies on several different flours, all found either at your local market; health food store; national chain stores like Whole Foods Market, Wild Oats, or Fresh Fields; or through the Internet. If you have to buy your flours online, be sure to check out the resources I have provided in this book, as they will save you time in searching for products.

This book is a cookbook, not a medical book. So I won't go into much detail about all of the medical conditions affected by consumption of gluten and gluten products. *Living Without* magazine offers wonderful articles and helpful information for those choosing a gluten-free diet. They also offer resources for finding great new products. That's where I found out about Gifts of Nature, Inc. a company certified to offer gluten-free oats.

I want to bring your attention to a few new gluten-free products on the market that I just love: hemp tortillas and brown rice tortillas. The hemp tortillas are chock full of protein (10 grams per serving), contain 8 grams of fiber, and provide omegas 3, 6, and 9 of healthy fat. The brand I use is called "Healthy Hemp." They are certified organic and are made by French Meadow Bakery, in Minneapolis, Minnesota. Their Web site is www.healthyhempbread.com. Trader Joe's carries brown rice tortillas, and they are great, too. They can be found at your local Trader Joe's grocery store. Both of these products work well with the Yam and Black Bean Burritos, found on page 91.

As for other grains, I love Bob's Red Mill's flours. These are some that I have used:

▶ Garbanzo bean flour (high in protein, and very flavorful)
▶ Sorghum flour (mimics wheat flour the best)
▶ Buckwheat flour (great for pancakes or waffles—a totally different grain from wheat)
▶ Millet flour (very light in flavor, contains same amount of protein as wheat flour)
▶ Tapioca flour (use in combination with other flours to produce light baked goods)
▶ Teff flour (use in cookies or cakes. Not great by itself, best if combined with rice flour)
▶ Quinoa flour (very good source of protein, and works well in breads, cakes, etc.)

Listed below are ideas of how to use these and other flours.

■ White Rice Flour

White rice flour is a grainy, bland flour that is milled from polished white rice. It works best in combination with other flours, such as potato, buckwheat, or corn flour. It can be used in cakes, breads, and cookies. It stores well (I store mine in the refrigerator to keep it fresh, but it is not required). There are different textures of white rice flour. The most common texture is fine, but regular is also available in health food stores. I haven't used this flour in any of the recipes in this book, but you may want to try it in combination with other flours.

■ Brown Rice Flour

I use this flour for many of my recipes. I like it because it contains more nutrients than the white variety. It is milled from unpolished brown rice. It has a nutty taste, and I use it in muffins and cookies. I also use it for my cobblers, and Marion Berry Bars. I store this flour in the refrigerator, as it contains oil, and has a shorter life span. It is also great combined with other flours such as sorghum, millet, buckwheat, or almond meal.

■ Garbanzo Bean and Other Legume-Based Flours

I use garbanzo bean and lentil flours for cookies. They can also be added to other flours (rice for instance) quite successfully. These flours offset the grainy texture of the rice flour and give it a nice flavor. These flours make good thickeners as well. I don't use them often, as they are strong in flavor, but I recommend you experiment with them. They do not need to be stored in the refrigerator.

■ Buckwheat Flour

Buckwheat flour is a member of the rhubarb family. It is not related to wheat. It is not even a grain. It is rich in iron, vitamin B, and calcium. It has a strong grainy flavor and is best used in waffles, pancakes, breads, and noodles (also look for cream of buckwheat and the various grinds of buckwheat groats, which make wonderful hot cereals, as well as wonderful side and main dishes).

■ Quinoa Flour

Quinoa (pronounced "keen-wa") flour is high in protein, contains twenty amino acids, including the ten "essential amino acids." It also contains vitamins A, C, D, B_1, B_2, E, and folic acid, niacin, calcium, iron, and phosphorus. It is used in cookies, pies, cakes, and pasta. It has a light, pleasant taste and works well combined with other flours.

■ Almond Meal Flour

Almond meal flour is comprised of blanched almonds that have been finely ground. It adds a rich, buttery flavor to cookies, muffins, cakes, and other desserts. It is a great source of protein, rich in fiber, vitamin E, and magnesium. It can also be used for breading. It should be stored in the refrigerator.

■ Tapioca Flour

Tapioca flour is also called tapioca starch, so if you are searching for it in the store, don't be dismayed if you can't find tapioca flour. I went to two stores before I figured out they were the same thing. It is derived from an exotic root and is also sold in granular and pearl forms for puddings and for pie thickeners. I do not use this as a flour alone, as it is very gummy, but combine it with other flours to provide a chewy texture. Tapioca mixed with brown or white rice flour and potato flour make wonderful flour. Do not attempt to make pizza dough out of this combination, though. I did and it bombed!

■ Potato Flour

Potato flour and potato starch are confusing terms. Unlike tapioca, above, the two are not alike: Potato flour is made from cooked potatoes. Potato starch is made from raw potatoes. This flour combines well with rice flours.

■ Sorghum Flour

Sorghum is another gluten-free flour that is very easy to work with. It is one of the main food crops used in India and Africa and is attracting a huge following in the United States for those with a gluten intolerance. Sorghum flour is high in soluble fiber and tastes very similar to wheat. When baking with sorghum flour, you will need to add xanthan gum ($1/2$ teaspoon per cup) to bind it together. It is great in cookies, piecrusts, cakes, and so on. You will see that I use it in several recipes. I encourage you to try it, too!

■ Soy Flour

I don't use this flour very often, as it has a strong flavor, but if you use small amounts and combine it with other flours, such as rice or millet, I am sure it would be fine. By itself, it just overpowers other ingredients. It does not store well, so buy it in small quantities and keep it in the refrigerator.

There are many other flours to choose from, including arrowroot flour, corn flour, teff, and nut and seed flours. I would encourage you to give them a try. All of these flours can be frozen. Rice flours last longer if you keep them in the refrigerator after opening.

FOODS TO AVOID IF ON A GLUTEN-FREE DIET

These foods are considered "not safe" for those adhering to a gluten-free diet.

- ▶ Ale and beer, malt, brewer's yeast
- ▶ Any kind of wheat flour, wheat germ, graham flour, bran, couscous, bulgur wheat, semolina
- ▶ Kamut, spelt, rye, barley
- ▶ Pasta, noodles, or dumplings containing any of the above grains (look for rice, corn, and other substitutes)
- ▶ Baked goods and cereals containing any of the above grains
- ▶ Canned meats, cold cuts, hot dogs (unless guaranteed pure meat), gravies
- ▶ Soy sauce and teriyaki sauce (unless labeled wheat-free)
- ▶ Textured vegetable protein (TVP)
- ▶ Food starch
- ▶ Crackers, bread crumbs, pretzels

For a complete list of "forbidden foods" please visit the Celiac Web site www.celiac.com. They provide a list of safe and forbidden foods that you can download and print. It is very helpful when just learning about which foods contain gluten and which do not.

OTHER INGREDIENTS

■ Millet

Millet is a grain rich in protein and minerals. It is easy to cook with and is good in stews, soups, as cereal, or in breads.

■ Arrowroot and Cornstarch

I prefer arrowroot to cornstarch, so that's all I use in this cookbook. So many people have allergies to corn, myself included, so I started using arrowroot and found that it works well for me. If you use cornstarch, be sure to mix it in a small amount of liquid before adding it to your sauce, as it can develop clumps. I recommend you whisk it thoroughly before adding it in with the rest of the ingredients Heat until it boils, then lower the heat and cook until thick.

Arrowroot can be mixed ahead with a small amount of liquid to thicken a recipe or it can be added directly to the rest of the ingredients. It will thicken without lumps. Don't boil arrowroot for too long, as it can break down and you will lose the thickness you desire. I turn up the heat, then lower it to a simmer rather than letting the mixture boil for a long period of time.

■ Baking Soda

I use baking soda in conjunction with baking powder, as it, alone, will not cause a product to leaven. I use it quite frequently in biscuits, cookies, and the like. It is best if you sift it with the flour and baking powder, as it is somewhat lumpy.

■ Baking Powder

If you are concerned about the health risks of aluminum, you can buy aluminum-free baking powder in health food stores. Ener-G Foods makes a gluten-free baking powder. I use baking powder frequently in my recipes, especially for cakes, cookies, bars, breads, and muffins.

■ Nuts and Seeds

I use nuts in many of my recipes; I frequently use almonds, cashews, walnuts, and Brazil nuts. I am also quite fond of pine nuts, so you see them in several of the recipes, too. Nuts are a great source of protein and healthy fats. However, if you have a nut allergy, be sure to read through the ingredients list of a recipe, before you begin to prepare it, to be sure it does not contain nuts of any kind.

I also like the health benefits of pumpkin seeds, sunflower seeds, and sesame seeds, and so I use them in many recipes as well. People who cannot eat tree nuts may be able to use these. Try substituting seeds for nuts. Be creative!

I love crunch in the foods I eat, so often I will add nuts or seeds simply to add more "crunch." The wonderful thing about nuts and seeds is that they are easy to find, and you can use them not only to bake with or in salads but you can also sprout them or use them to make very tasty milks. See the recipe for almond milk, found on page 158.

COOKING GUIDE FOR GRAINS

IF YOU ARE unused to using the following grains, here is a guide to their preparation:

■ Quinoa

To prepare quinoa, you want to start by rinsing it very well. Place it in a colander or small strainer (the seeds are very small so a regular-size colander will not work), run cold water over the quinoa, and drain. Quinoa cooks fairly quickly. To cook 1 cup of dry quinoa you will want to add it to 2 cups of water or vegetable stock. Bring it to a boil, then lower the heat to a simmer and cover. The quinoa should be ready in about 20 minutes. This will yield about 3½ cups of cooked quinoa. If your recipe does not call for this much quinoa, no worries, you will find many ways to use the leftovers. I love it in salads, soups, stews, and stuffed into bell peppers!

■ Millet

Rinse 1 cup of millet and drain, then place in a pan with 2½ cups of water. Add a pinch of salt if you wish, and you can also use vegetable stock in place of water, or cut the amount to half water, half vegetable stock. The cooking method is the same as for quinoa: bring to a boil, then lower the heat and simmer, covered, until light and fluffy. This grain is very small and light, but it takes 25 to 30 minutes to cook. This amount of millet will yield about 3½ cups cooked millet.

■ Oats

There are varying times for the different types of oats. For example, steel-cut oats will need to cook for about 45 minutes. So, if you begin with 1 cup of gluten-free steel-cut oats, place them in a pan with 3 cups of water and bring to a boil. Lower the heat and simmer until done, about 1 hour.

If you are using gluten-free rolled oats, however, place 2 cups of water in a pan and heat to a boil with 1 cup of rolled oats. Lower the heat and simmer until done, about 15 minutes. This will yield about 1½ cups of cooked oatmeal.

■ Brown Rice

To prepare brown, or what I prefer to use, "red" rice (Lundberg Family Farms has a wonderful variety of brown rice, Wehani, that is actually red in color), rinse 1 cup of brown rice and drain, then add to a pan along with 2 cups of water or vegetable stock. Bring to a boil, then lower the heat to medium-low, cover, and simmer until done, 45 to 50 minutes. Add a pinch of salt to the cooking water if you wish, or other herbs, too, such as rosemary or thyme. This recipe will yield about 3 cups of rice.

■ Wild Rice

To prepare wild rice, wash 1 cup well and place it in a pan with 3 cups of water. Bring it to a boil, then lower the heat, cover, and simmer until done, 55 to 60 minutes. This amount of rice will yield about 4 cups cooked.

■ Polenta (Cornmeal)

Place 1 cup of coarse cornmeal in a pan with 3 cups (if you like it wetter, use $3\frac{1}{2}$ cups) of water or milk (I prefer it made with milk), and add a pinch of salt. Bring to a boil, then lower the heat, cover, and cook for 20 to 25 minutes. This will make about $2\frac{1}{2}$ cups.

THE
RECIPES

APPETIZERS

APPLE SALSA

BLACK BEAN SALSA

CURRIED BEAN DIP

GUACAMOLE

HUMMUS

MAPLE CANDIED NUTS

SALSA

SPICY MIXED NUTS AND SEEDS

APPLE SALSA

This salsa can be served with veggies or corn chips or used as a topping for pancakes. I think it would even work on top of a roasted yam. Yum!

- 3 tart apples (including Granny Smith and Gala, or all of one kind)
- 3 tablespoons agave nectar or brown rice syrup
- 2–3 tablespoons fresh lime juice
- ½ cup chopped fresh cilantro
- ½ cup chopped walnuts, almonds, cashews, or macadamia nuts
- ½ teaspoon ground cinnamon

■ Peel the apples (or not, if you prefer), core them, and dice them into small pieces. (You can use a food processor to dice them.) Place in a large bowl with the rest of the ingredients. Mix together well and chill.

BLACK BEAN SALSA

Another favorite recipe, *this is quick to fix, full of protein and good flavor, and goes well with any Mexican-style meal or by itself as a dip served with chips. You can also add avocado to this recipe, or red pinto beans in place of the black beans.*

1 (15-ounce can) black beans, drained and rinsed

1 small jalapeño, seeded and chopped finely

1 medium-size red bell pepper, seeded and chopped

1 small red onion, chopped finely

1 clove garlic, chopped

2 cups diced or chopped tomatoes

¼ cup orange juice, freshly squeezed if possible

1 tablespoon olive oil

¼ cup lime juice, freshly squeezed if possible

■ Mix all of the ingredients in a large bowl and stir to blend everything together. Place, covered, in the refrigerator until chilled.

CURRIED BEAN DIP

This is a great appetizer for a party. Serve with veggies or chips and watch it fly out of the bowl!

1 (15-ounce can) garbanzo beans, drained and rinsed

1 (15-ounce can) white kidney beans, drained and rinsed

¼ cup olive oil

1 teaspoon curry powder

1 teaspoon ground cumin

2 tablespoons lemon juice, freshly squeezed if possible

½ cup chopped fresh cilantro

Pinch of red pepper flakes

¼ teaspoon sea salt

Freshly ground pepper

■ Place all of the ingredients into a food processor or blender, and blend until smooth. Adjust seasonings, cover, and chill for a few hours to really let the flavors blend together. Serve with cut vegetables or chips.

GUACAMOLE

I often add Roma tomatoes to this recipe. It is wonderful served with the J&J's Black Bean and Yam Burritos (page 91). Served by itself with chips, it won't last long, I can guarantee it.

2½ cups peeled and mashed avocado (2 large avocados)

1 tablespoon Tofutti soy sour cream (optional)

1 clove garlic, minced

⅓ cup seeded and finely chopped red bell pepper

1 small jalapeño, seeded and chopped finely

½ cup chopped fresh cilantro

¼ teaspoon ground cumin

Juice of 1 lime

Pinch of red pepper flakes

Salt and freshly ground pepper

■ Place the mashed avocados into a large bowl. Add the rest of the ingredients and stir together well, seasoning to taste with salt and pepper. Cover and chill before serving.

HUMMUS

I love hummus. It is full of protein and has such a warm, inviting flavor. This is wonderful served at a party, with chips or vegetables on the side, or spread over apples for a quick snack. It is also a terrific healthy snack stuffed in celery for your children.

2 (15-ounce) cans garbanzo beans (chickpeas), drained and rinsed (reserve liquid)

5–6 tablespoons lemon juice, freshly squeezed

⅓ cup sesame tahini (or more if desired)

2 cloves garlic, minced finely

½ teaspoon sea salt

Freshly ground pepper

Pinch of cayenne

Olive oil

■ Place the garbanzo beans, lemon juice, tahini, and garlic in a blender or food processor. Blend until smooth. If the mixture is too thick, use the reserved liquid from the garbanzo beans and add a small amount, a little at a time, until the mixture blends smoothly. Remove from the blender and add the salt, pepper and cayenne. Place in a serving bowl and drizzle a small amount of olive oil on top. Serve with veggies.

MAPLE CANDIED NUTS

Well, what can I say about these? I can't keep them in the house, that's what! They are so good, I just keep eating them. So, my answer to that is to give them away: to put them in jars and tie with a ribbon as gifts. These nuts are great in the Spinach and Pear Salad (page 50) or as a garnish for any salad.

1½ cups raw walnuts or pecans
2 tablespoons pure maple syrup

■ Preheat the oven to 300°F. Toss the nuts in the maple syrup. Well, don't really "toss" them, place them in a bowl and pour the syrup over the nuts and stir to coat well. Spread out the nuts on a rimmed cookie sheet or jelly-roll pan as evenly as you can, in a single layer. Roast them at 300°F until they are browned, but *not* burned. Check them during the roasting process and stir them several times while they are cooking. The nuts should be browned and ready to come out of the oven in 20 to 25 minutes. Once they are cooled, put them in an airtight container and keep them either at room temperature or in the refrigerator (where you won't see them as often).

SALSA

This recipe is so easy to make and it makes quite a bit. I keep it in the refrigerator for up to a week at a time. If you like more "heat," add some more cayenne or jalapeño. I made it "mild" so it wouldn't tip you over the edge!

1 cup seeded and chopped or sliced red bell pepper (roasted if you have it)

1 clove garlic, chopped finely

2 tablespoons finely chopped red onion

4 large Roma tomatoes, seeded and chopped

¼ cup chopped fresh cilantro, (or more if you prefer)

Juice of 1 large lime

¼ teaspoon coarse kosher salt

¼ teaspoon freshly ground pepper

¼ teaspoon ground cumin

¼ teaspoon organic apple cider (such as Bragg's)

1 jalapeño, seeded and sliced (optional)

Pinch of cayenne or red pepper flakes

■ Place all of the ingredients in a food processor or blender, and whirl until the consistency is that of salsa. If you prefer a chunkier salsa, process instead in brief on-and-off bursts until it is the texture you wish. I like my salsa quite fine, so I blend until the mixture is all of the same consistency, and then I adjust seasonings if needed (I like a lot of freshly ground pepper).

SPICY MIXED NUTS AND SEEDS

These make a good snack or can be used on top of salads to add protein and zip. They store well in an airtight container for several weeks.

1 cup pecans
½ cup sunflower seeds
¼ cup pumpkin seeds
½ cup walnuts
¼ cup almonds
2 tablespoons grapeseed oil
2 teaspoons chile powder
2 tablespoons agave nectar
1 teaspoon salt
Pinch of cayenne

■ Place all of the ingredients in a large bowl and mix well. Preheat the oven to 300°F and spread the ingredients on a large cookie sheet, in a single layer. Bake until toasted, stirring during the baking process at least once or twice, 20 to 25 minutes. Cool and store in an airtight container.

SOUPS

BRUCE'S FAVORITE CURRIED APPLE AND CAULIFLOWER SOUP

CORN CHOWDER

FAVA BEAN AND VEGETABLE SOUP

FRESH AVOCADO AND CUCUMBER SOUP

HOMEMADE VEGETABLE STOCK

MEDITERRANEAN SOUP

MINESTRONE SOUP

RICE AND VEGETABLE SOUP

ROASTED TOMATO SOUP

THAI VEGETABLE SOUP

TOMATO AND WHITE BEAN SOUP

BRUCE'S FAVORITE CURRIED APPLE AND CAULIFLOWER SOUP

SERVES 4

Typically, this sort of soup would be pureed, but I didn't do that. I like to see the apple and cauliflower in this soup, so I left it just as it is. Obviously Bruce, the owner of Whole Foods Market in Gig Harbor liked it just the way it is, too.

2 tablespoons olive or coconut oil

2 cups chopped sweet onions, such as Vidalia

4 cups (1 head or about 1½ pounds) coarsely chopped organic cauliflower florets

2 cloves garlic, chopped

2 cups cored and diced apple

1 cup chopped walnuts

1 teaspoon curry powder

½ teaspoon ground turmeric

1 (32-ounce) carton organic vegetable stock, or homemade (4 cups) (page 34)

2 cups water, or 1 cup water and 1 cup white wine

1 tablespoon agave nectar

1 cup chopped fresh cilantro

Sea salt and freshly ground pepper

■ Heat the oil in a 3- to 4-quart stockpot over medium-high heat and add the onions and cauliflower. Sauté until the onion is soft and cauliflower is crisp-tender. Add the garlic, apples, walnuts, curry powder, and turmeric, and continue to cook for 4 to 5 minutes. Add the vegetable stock, water (and wine, if using), agave nectar, and cilantro. Lower the heat to medium-low and simmer until the vegetables are fork tender. Add the salt and pepper to taste, and serve.

CORN CHOWDER

I really love corn chowder and it's perfect served alongside a big garden salad. If you don't want to use butternut squash, or you don't have any, simply increase the potatoes and enjoy. You can also add yams or sweet potatoes in place of the squash, if you prefer.

1 tablespoon olive oil

1 leek, chopped (white part only)

1 small onion

2 cups peeled, seeded, and diced butternut squash

2 red potatoes, scrubbed, peeled, and cubed

2 cloves garlic

1 (15-ounce can) light coconut milk

2 cups frozen or fresh white or yellow corn

2 small bay leaves

¼ cup chopped fresh parsley

¼ teaspoon ground cumin

1 cup water

1 teaspoon sea salt

¼–½ teaspoon freshly ground black pepper

■ Heat the oil in a large stockpot. When the oil is hot, add the leek, onion, and butternut squash. Cook for 4 to 5 minutes over medium heat. Add the potatoes and garlic, and continue to cook until the potatoes and squash are beginning to soften, 6 to 10 minutes. If the veggies stick to the bottom of the pot, add a drip of oil. Add the coconut milk, corn, bay leaves, parsley, cumin, and water. Simmer, covered, until flavors blend and the potatoes and squash are cooked through but not mushy. Season with salt and fresh ground pepper. If you prefer your chowder thinner, add a little more water.

FAVA BEAN AND VEGETABLE SOUP

Fava beans are so full of flavor and, mixed with summer vegetables, you can't go wrong. You can also add some diced tomato, if you wish. Don't forget to clean the leeks really well, as dirt collects in its leaves and, unless you rinse it thoroughly, you will be sorry!

1 tablespoon olive oil

2 large leeks (white part only), cleaned, or 1 large red onion

½ cup chopped baby carrots

2 cups shelled fresh fava beans (see Note)

1 cup ends trimmed, cut into bite-size pieces fresh asparagus

1 cup cooked, chopped green beans

3 cloves garlic, chopped

1 (32-ounce) carton organic vegetable stock, or 4 cups homemade (page 34)

½ cup white wine

¾ cup chopped fresh basil

Kosher salt

Freshly ground pepper

Fresh parsley, for garnish (optional)

■ In a large Dutch oven or stockpot, heat the oil over medium-high heat and add the leeks. Sauté until they become soft, 3 to 4 minutes. Add the carrots, fava beans, and asparagus, and continue cooking for another 4 to 5 minutes. Add the cooked green beans and garlic, and sauté for 1 minute. Add the vegetable stock, wine, and basil, and lower the heat to low. Simmer until the beans are cooked, and the flavors have blended. Season to taste with salt and pepper. Garnish with parsley, if desired.

> Note: In rare cases, fava beans can cause a fatal allergic reaction (a disease called "favism") in some people of African, Mediterranean, or Southeast Asian descent.

FRESH AVOCADO AND CUCUMBER SOUP

This soup is light, creamy, and, because it contains cucumber, very refreshing. I think summer is the best time of year for this soup, as cucumbers are at their very best then. I do hope you shop for your cucmbers at your local organic produce farms.

1 cup soy or hemp milk

4 green onions, chopped

2 large avocados, peeled, pitted, and cut into chunks

Juice of ½ lime (or more if desired)

¼ teaspoon sea salt

1 large cucumber, peeled and chopped

¼ cup chopped fresh cilantro

Freshly cracked pepper

Pinch of cayenne (optional)

■ Place all of the ingredients except the pepper in a food processor or blender, and puree until the mixture is well blended, with a very smooth consistency. Add the pepper and adjust seasonings. You can also add a pinch of cayenne if you want more of a "kick" to the soup. Chill before serving.

HOMEMADE VEGETABLE STOCK

It's easier to buy organic vegetable stock at the grocery store, but they all include so much sodium that I wanted to share my recipe with you. You can use this broth for many of the recipes that call for vegetable stock. Feel free to use whatever vegetables you have in the refrigerator. Vegetable stock is very versatile. There is no "right" way to make it, so be creative.

1 tablespoon organic extra-virgin olive oil

1 large red onion, peeled and cut into quarters

2 large carrots, cut into chunks

4 small potatoes, scrubbed and cut into halves or quarters

1 small yam, peeled and cut into quarters

2 cups washed and chopped spinach

4–5 cloves garlic, peeled and ends cut off

8 cups purified water

2 large bay leaves

¼ cup chopped fresh parsley

1 teaspoon coarse kosher salt

½ teaspoon freshly ground pepper, or more to taste

1 (12-ounce) can whole or diced organic tomatoes

- Heat a large stockpot over medium-high heat and pour in the olive oil. Add the onion, carrots, potatoes, and yam, and sauté for 4 to 5 minutes. Add the spinach and garlic, and continue to cook for 3 to 4 minutes. Add the water, bay leaves, parsley, salt, pepper, tomatoes, and any other herbs you like, and lower the heat to low. Simmer for a few hours, or longer if you prefer.
- You can now do one of two things: (1) puree this mixture in a blender or food processor until completely smooth, and use as a stock (you will need to add more water to it); or (2) strain out and discard all the vegetables and use the remaining stock for soups, stews, and risottos.

MEDITERRANEAN SOUP

SERVES 4

I try to add protein to every meal, so I tend to include beans and nuts in many of the recipes in this book. The wonderful thing about the Mediterranean diet is that people of that region always use beans and vegetables in their recipes. If you want more "substance" in this soup, add one cup of cooked brown rice or quinoa.

1 large red onion, chopped

2 large carrots, peeled and sliced

1–2 tablespoons olive oil

3 cloves garlic, chopped or minced

1 (32-ounce) carton organic vegetable stock, or 4 cups homemade (page 34)

2 bay leaves

1 teaspoon dried thyme

2 tablespoons dried parsley, or ¼ cup chopped fresh

1 (15-ounce) can white kidney beans (cannellini beans), drained and rinsed

½ cup red or white wine (preferably red)

1 (6-ounce) can tomato sauce

Salt and pepper

- In a 3-quart stockpot, sauté the onion and carrots in the oil over medium heat for 4 to 5 minutes. Add the garlic and continue to sauté, until the carrots are tender. Add the vegetable stock, bay leaves, thyme, parsley, kidney beans, wine, and tomato sauce. Simmer over medium-low heat until the flavors blend, about 30 minutes. Season with salt and pepper, and serve.

MINESTRONE SOUP

This hearty soup will warm you all the way through to your bones. It is full of flavor and texture. Add 1 cup of mushrooms if you desire.

1 tablespoon olive oil

1 large red onion, chopped

3 stalks celery, chopped

½ cup chopped carrots

1 green bell pepper, seeded and chopped (about 1 cup)

1 medium-size zucchini, chopped

5–6 cloves garlic, chopped

1 (15-ounce) can red kidney beans, drained and rinsed

1 (15-ounce can) white kidney beans (cannellini beans), drained and rinsed

1 (32-ounce) carton organic vegetable stock, or 4 cups homemade (page 34)

1 (14-ounce) can diced tomatoes

2 cups tomato sauce

½ cup chopped fresh parsley

½ cup chopped fresh basil

1 teaspoon dried tarragon

1 teaspoon dried oregano

2 tablespoons wheat-free tamari sauce

1 tablespoon balsamic vinegar

1½ cups cooked brown or wild rice

Pinch of red pepper flakes

Salt and pepper

■ In a large stockpot, heat the oil over medium-high heat. Add the onions and sauté until soft, 4 to 5 minutes. Add the celery, carrots, green bell pepper, and zucchini, and sauté for another 6 to 8 minutes. If the vegetables start to stick to the bottom of the pot, instead of adding more oil, add a little bit of the vegetable stock, and continue to sauté. Add the garlic and cook for 1 to 2 minutes. Add the beans, vegetable stock, tomatoes, tomato sauce, herbs, tamari sauce, vinegar, and cooked rice. Simmer until the vegetables are tender and flavors have blended, about 30 minutes. Add the red pepper flakes, salt, and pepper to taste, and serve. If soup is too thick, add a bit more vegetable stock or water.

RICE AND VEGETABLE SOUP

This is a very hearty soup. It will fill you up and stick to your ribs for quite some time. I gave my friend James some of this soup, and he feasted on it for several days. He loved it. It makes a lot, but you can freeze it if you can't eat it up quickly.

1 cup Lundberg Family Farms Wehani & Wild Rice Medley or another wild rice mixture (do not use instant rice!)

¼ teaspoon salt, or to taste

½ teaspoon herbes de Provence

3 cups chopped broccoli, several florets reserved for garnish

1–2 tablespoons olive oil

1 large onion, chopped

3 large celery stalks, chopped

1 large carrot, chopped

2 cloves garlic, chopped

1 cup washed and chopped spinach

1½ (32-ounce) cartons organic vegetable stock, or 6 cups homemade (page 34)

1 tablespoon wheat-free tamari sauce

1 tablespoon chopped fresh parsley

¼ teaspoon freshly ground pepper

¼ teaspoon red pepper flakes (optional)

- Place the rice in a 2-quart saucepan and cover with 2 cups of water. Add a pinch of salt and the herbes de Provence. Bring the water to a boil, then lower the heat to low or medium-low, and simmer until rice is cooked, about 50 minutes. Remove the lid, fluff the rice, and set aside to cool.

- In the meantime, steam the chopped broccoli and set aside, reserving the broccoli florets to use as a garnish later. Heat a stockpot over medium-high heat and heat 1 tablespoon of the olive oil. Sauté the onion, celery, carrots, and garlic for about 5 minutes. Stir occasionally while cooking. Add the spinach and continue to cook for 2 to 3 minutes. Lower the heat and add the vegetable stock, steamed broccoli, and cooked rice. Simmer for 5 to 10 minutes, or until the vegetables are tender.

- Place small batches of the soup in a blender or food processor, and puree until smooth. Continue this process until all of the soup has been blended. Return mixture to the stockpot and add the tamari sauce, parsley, red pepper flakes, and salt and pepper to taste. Add the remaining broccoli florets and serve.

ROASTED TOMATO SOUP

I hated tomato soup as a kid. You know most people bought that brand that I won't say, and it really wasn't soup anyway. This is soup, and I hope you like it as much as I do. I am a convert now.

6 large tomatoes, cut in half

5 cloves garlic, peeled and cut in half

Salt and pepper

1 tablespoon olive oil

1 large onion or 1–2 well-washed leeks (white part only), chopped

1 large red bell pepper, seeded and chopped

2 small carrots, chopped

1 (32-ounce) carton organic vegetable stock, or 4 cups homemade (page 34)

¼ cup chopped fresh basil

■ Preheat the oven to 400°F and layer the tomatoes and garlic on a large, lightly oiled cookie sheet (with sides). Sprinkle with salt and pepper, and roast until soft, 45 to 50 minutes. (Keep an eye on the garlic, it may be ready before the tomatoes. You will need to remove the cloves from the oven if they are cooked before the tomatoes are ready to come out.) Let cool, then remove the skin of the tomatoes.

■ Meanwhile, sauté the onions in a small saucepan with 1 tbs. of olive oil. When the onions begin to soften, add the bell pepper and continue to sauté until peppers are soft. Simmer the carrots in a 2-quart stockpot, in the vegetable stock. Add the cooked onions and peppers, the tomatoes and garlic after they have roasted. Bring to a boil. Add the basil and lower the heat to low. Simmer for 5 to 10 minutes. Puree this mixture in a food processor or blender until smooth. You may want to do this a little at a time if you are using a blender. If the mixture is too thick, add a small amount of water to thin it (no more than 1 cup). Return the soup to the stockpot, season to taste, and heat through.

THAI VEGETABLE SOUP

SERVES 6

I was visiting Port Townsend, Washington, one weekend and came across this wonderful little place where I had lunch. The soup that day was something like this. I enjoyed it so much I wrote down as many of the ingredients as I could identify and then came home and tried to reproduce it. I know it's not their recipe, but it's as close as I could get. It is very good, and I hope you enjoy it.

1 cup chopped red onion

1 tablespoon olive oil

2 large carrots, chopped

1 small zucchini, chopped

1 red or yellow bell pepper, seeded and chopped

1½ cups cleaned and stemmed shiitaki or cremini mushrooms

2 cups chopped Savoy cabbage

4 cloves garlic, chopped

1 tablespoon finely chopped jalapeño (optional)

1 (14-ounce) can light coconut milk

14 ounces water (measure in coconut milk can), or more if desired (I like my soups thick)

2 tablespoons wheat-free tamari sauce

Juice of ½ lime

1 tablespoon red chile paste

Pinch of red pepper flakes

¼ cup chopped fresh cilantro

Pinch each of cumin, turmeric, and cardamom

Freshly ground pepper

Coarse kosher salt

■ In a large stockpot, sauté the onion in the olive oil for 4 to 5 minutes over medium heat. Add the carrots, zucchini, and bell pepper, and continue to cook for another 2 to 3 minutes. Add the mushrooms, cabbage, garlic, and jalapeño, and continue to cook until the veggies are fork tender, 5 to 6 minutes. Add the coconut milk, water, tamari sauce, lime juice, chile paste, red pepper flakes, cilantro, and spices, and simmer to blend the flavors, 20 to 30 minutes over low heat. Adjust the seasonings, if desired. Be sure to add some freshly ground pepper just before serving.

TOMATO AND WHITE BEAN SOUP

Here is another take on tomato soup. This one has more protein and also a different flavor. It stores well in the refrigerator and is great to take to work or school for lunch.

1½ tablespoons olive oil

1 cup chopped onion

4 cloves garlic, chopped

½ cup roasted and chopped red bell pepper

¼ teaspoon fennel seeds

1 (15-ounce) can white kidney beans (cannellini beans), drained and rinsed

1 (28-ounce) can organic diced or chopped tomatoes

1½ cups vegetable stock (store-bought or homemade, page 34)

1 cup white wine

2 bay leaves

6 tablespoons chopped fresh basil

1 tablespoon dried parsley

Pinch of red pepper flakes

Freshly ground pepper

Coarse kosher salt

■ In a stockpot, heat the oil over medium heat. Add the onion and sauté until soft, 5 to 6 minutes. Add the garlic and continue to sauté for 1 minute. Add the roasted bell peppers and fennel seeds, and sauté for 2 to 3 minutes. Add the white beans, tomatoes, stock, white wine, bay leaves, and herbs, and lower the heat to low. Simmer until the flavors are well blended and the soup is heated through, 20 to 30 minutes. Season to taste with red pepper flakes, salt, and pepper, and serve.

SALADS

BETCHA BY GOLLY BEAN SALAD

CARROT SALAD

CUCUMBER SALAD

FRUIT AND NUT SALAD

GARDEN SALAD

MEXICAN QUINOA SALAD

MOCK TABBOULEH SALAD

QUINOA AND VEGETABLE SALAD

SPINACH AND PEAR SALAD

SUPER ANTIOXIDANT SALAD

SWEET POTATO SALAD

WALDORF SALAD

ZIPPITY DO DA COLESLAW

BETCHA BY GOLLY BEAN SALAD

Beans are a great source of protein, and bean salads at a summer picnic are a must! Try this one. I have used three different types of beans, and added walnuts for crunch and a dose of healthy fats. Cilantro is one of my favorite herbs, and I put quite a bit into this recipe. If you don't care for cilantro, substitute parsley.

1 (15-ounce) can black beans, drained and rinsed

1 (15-ounce) can kidney beans, drained and rinsed

1 (15-ounce) can white kidney beans (cannellini beans, drained and rinsed

1–2 tablespoons orange juice, preferably freshly squeezed

2 cloves garlic, chopped finely

½ cup finely chopped red bell pepper

1 small red onion or 2 shallots, chopped finely

½ cup chopped walnuts

¼ cup chopped fresh cilantro, or 1 tablespoon dried

¼ teaspoon toasted cumin seeds

Salt and freshly ground pepper (optional)

■ Place all the ingredients in a large mixing bowl and stir to combine well. Be sure to mix in the orange juice well so the flavors really come together. Cover and place in the refrigerator until chilled. Season with salt and pepper, if desired.

CARROT SALAD

This salad not only tastes great, it looks lovely. If you use soy sour cream in place of the vegan mayonnaise, it will give the salad a slightly sweeter taste. This salad stores well in the refrigerator for several days.

6 carrots, peeled and grated

½ cup chopped walnuts, pecans, macadamia nuts, cashews, or almonds

½ cup currants or raisins (golden raisins look nice in this salad)

1 tablespoon finely chopped green onion

1 tablespoon sunflower, poppy, or sesame seeds

2 tablespoons vegan mayonnaise

Juice of ½ lemon

Sea salt and freshly ground pepper

■ In a large bowl, combine the carrots, walnuts, currants, green onion, and sunflower seeds, and toss well. In a small bowl, whisk together the mayonnaise and lemon juice. Pour over the vegetables and stir well. If you prefer more dressing, increase the amount of mayonnaise and lemon juice. Season to taste with salt and pepper.

CUCUMBER SALAD

Cucumbers are so refreshing. I love them in salads, and this one really has a kick to it. If it is too spicy for you, use less apple cider and go easy on the pepper. I like it like this, and I hope you do, too.

Dressing

- ¼ cup apple cider vinegar (I recommend Bragg's)
- 2 tablespoons grapeseed or canola oil
- ¼ teaspoon fresh cracked pepper, or more to taste
- ¼ teaspoon sea salt
- 2 teaspoons organic sugar

- 2 medium-size cucumbers, peeled and sliced
- 1 large red onion, sliced very thinly
- 2 large tomatoes, seeded and cut into bite-size pieces

■ Whisk together in a large bowl all the dressing ingredients, then add the cucumbers, onion, and tomatoes, and stir to blend all the flavors together. Place in the refrigerator to chill thoroughly before serving.

FRUIT AND NUT SALAD

This is the *kind of salad that you can throw just about anything in and it will be wonderful. Summer is a time to enjoy fresh fruits, so be creative and add cantaloupe or other melons, grapes, whatever you like to this; just add more lime or lemon juice and toss.*

½ cup chopped walnuts

1 large organic apple, cored and chopped

3–4 dried figs, chopped

2–3 Medjool dates, pitted and chopped

1 large organic orange, cut into bite-size pieces

5 large organic strawberries, hulled, and cut into quarters, plus 2 hulled strawberries to use for the dressing

½ cup chopped mango

1 large organic banana, peeled and cut into bite-size pieces

2 tablespoons pine nuts

1 teaspoon sesame seeds

Juice of 1 lime

■ Put all of the chopped and sliced fruits and nuts into a large salad bowl. Place the lime juice and the 2 extra strawberries in a blender and blend together. Pour over the salad and toss.

GARDEN SALAD

This salad is full of great vegetables and fruits, but I don't want you to limit yourself to just these ingredients. Add some carrots, cauliflower, or broccoli, if you wish. This is my favorite green salad, but I change it up as the season provides various vegetables. I can't even count the times I made this last summer, but each time I made it, I prepared it slightly differently. For example, I added snow peas from the garden, I added spinach, I used raspberries or strawberries instead of blueberries. It is so versatile. Try dressing with Balsamic Salad Dressing (page 170) or Raspberry Vinaigrette (page 177), or just add oil and vinegar. Or squeeze on some lemon juice and a dash of olive oil, and you are good to go! Enjoy.

4 cups chopped romaine hearts

1 large avocado, peeled, pitted, and chopped

1 large Roma tomato, chopped

1 large red bell pepper, seeded and chopped

6–7 kalamata olives, pitted and chopped

½ cup blueberries

¼ cup pine nuts

1 large pear, cored and chopped

1 small cucumber, peeled and chopped

½ cup chopped carrots

■ Place all of the ingredients in a large bowl. Add your favorite salad dressing and toss. Serve immediately.

MEXICAN QUINOA SALAD

For this satisfying quinoa salad, I have taken you south of the border. There is so much you can do with this recipe. If you are in the mood, add some avocado or roasted corn.

1½ cups water

1 cup quinoa, rinsed with cold water and drained

½ cup seeded and chopped red or yellow bell peppers

1 small jalapeño, seeded and diced finely (optional)

1 small red onion, or 2 green onions, chopped fine

2 Roma tomatoes, chopped

1 (15-ounce) can pinto or other beans (such as red kidney or black), drained and rinsed

½ teaspoon ground cumin

¼ cup fresh cilantro, chopped (optional)

½ cup salsa (page 26)

1 tablespoon canola oil

Juice of 1 lime

Freshly ground pepper

Sea salt

■ Heat the water to boiling in a 2-quart saucepan and add the quinoa. Lower the heat to medium-low and cover. Cook until the liquid is absorbed, 15 to 20 minutes. Remove from the heat and cool.

■ When the quinoa has cooled, add the peppers, onions, tomatoes, beans, cumin, cilantro, salsa, oil, and lime juice. Season with the pepper and salt, and toss to blend well. Chill before serving.

MOCK TABBOULEH SALAD

SERVES 4

This is another summer salad. You can make it anytime of year, really, but I think of it as a summer salad because of the fresh mint, tomatoes, green onions, and so on. All of these vegetables are at their freshest in the summer, so it just feels best to make it then. If you live someplace where you have summer all year long, you are very lucky!

6–7 kalamata olives (or black olives), chopped

3–4 small green onions or leeks, chopped

1 small red bell pepper, seeded and chopped

2 large tomatoes, chopped

3 tablespoons chopped fresh mint

¼ cup chopped fresh parsley

1 cup quinoa, cooked and cooled (see previous recipe)

Juice of 1 lemon

3 tablespoons olive oil

¼ teaspoon salt

Freshly ground pepper

■ Place the olives, vegetables, and herbs in a large salad bowl. Add the cooled quinoa, lemon juice, and oil. Toss together. Season with salt and pepper, and chill before serving.

QUINOA AND VEGETABLE SALAD

Quinoa has such a soft, nutty flavor that it really is wonderful in salads. I like this salad because it combines everything into one meal: protein, carbohydrates, and healthy fats. I also love limes, so try lime juice in place of the lemon for a change.

½ cup chopped walnuts

1 cup chopped carrots

2 green onions, chopped fine

1 small yellow bell pepper, chopped

1 cup quinoa, cooked and cooled (page 47)

1 cup cooked, sliced green beans

½ cup cooked mushrooms (chanterelles or other varieties are fine)

Juice of 1 lemon

3 tablespoons canola oil

½ teaspoon fresh tarragon

½ teaspoon sea salt

Freshly ground pepper

■ Place the walnuts, all of the chopped vegetables, and the mushrooms in a large mixing bowl. Add the cooled quinoa and toss. In a small bowl, whisk together the lemon juice, oil, tarragon, salt, and pepper. Toss together with the quinoa mixture and adjust seasonings to taste. Chill prior to serving.

SPINACH AND PEAR SALAD

SERVES 4

I make this recipe just so I can eat the candied walnuts! It is really good.

- 4 cups washed and chopped baby spinach
- 1 cup Maple Candied Nuts (page 25)
- ¼ cup finely chopped red onion
- ½ cup seeded and chopped red bell pepper
- 2 large pears, cored and chopped (about 2 cups)
- Raspberry Vinaigrette (page 177) or Balsamic Salad Dressing (page 170)

■ Place all of the salad ingredients in a large bowl and toss with your preferred dressing. Chill and serve.

SUPER ANTIOXIDANT SALAD

This is truly exactly what its name says. It's a healthy salad that is good for you and tastes wonderful. Use fruits in season and add to them, if you wish. You don't need to use much vinaigrette; the fruits are so flavorful that you don't want to overpower them.

1 cup fresh blueberries

1 mango, pitted and chopped, or 1 cup frozen mango, thawed

1 cup seeded and sliced red bell pepper

2 cups coarsely chopped red cabbage

¼ cup chopped walnuts or other nuts

2 cups chopped romaine hearts

1 cup bite-size pieces of cantaloupe

Raspberry Vinaigrette (page 177)

■ Place all of the salad ingredients in a large bowl and toss together with a small amount of Raspberry Vinaigrette dressing.

SWEET POTATO SALAD

This is a different spin on traditional potato salad. I love yams and thought they have so much more flavor than potatoes that I decided to make a new version of an old favorite.

2 large garnet yams, peeled and cut into 1-inch-thick slices, then into chunks (about 6 cups)

½ cup finely chopped fennel

1 small zucchini, chopped

1 medium-size yellow or green bell pepper, seeded and chopped

3 stalks celery, chopped

¾ cup chopped carrot

1 (4-ounce) can black olives, drained

½ cup pine nuts, toasted

½–1 cup vegan mayonnaise

1 tablespoon dill, dried

2 tablespoons chopped fresh parsley

¼–½ cup (depending on your taste) organic apple cider vinegar (I like Bragg's)

Salt

Freshly ground pepper

■ Steam the yams until fork tender. Cool completely.

■ While yams are cooling, place the fennel, zucchini, bell pepper, celery, carrots, olives, and pine nuts in a large mixing bowl. Add the cooled yams and stir in the mayonnaise, dill, parsley, and vinegar.

■ Mix together until well blended and adjust the mayonnaise to your desired consistency. Add salt and pepper to taste. Refrigerate for at least 1 hour before serving.

WALDORF SALAD

I used to love Waldorf salad when I was a youngster, but it wasn't this version. I wanted to jazz up the old style of Waldorf salad, so I added quinoa, carrots, and dried cranberries. I hope you like my version better than the one Mom used to make (no offense to those moms who make the standard version!).

½ cup dried cranberries or raisins

3 large apples (organic Galas are my choice), peeled and cubed

½ cup chopped walnuts

2 stalks celery, chopped finely

2 medium-size carrots, grated or chopped

1½ cups quinoa, cooked and cooled (page 47)

⅓ cup Tofutti soy sour cream

2 tablespoons lemon juice

¼ teaspoon salt

Freshly ground pepper

■ Combine the cranberries, apples, walnuts, celery, and carrots in a large mixing bowl. Add the cooled quinoa. In a separate bowl, combine the soy sour cream and lemon juice, and mix together until well blended. Pour this mixture over the salad and toss to blend. Season with salt and pepper, and chill well before serving.

ZIPPITY DO DA COLESLAW

My taste testers thought it was odd that I added pineapple to this recipe, until they tried it. Then they changed their minds and didn't think it was so odd after all. This slaw is full of color, flavor, and lots of fiber. Take this along the next time you go to a friend's house for dinner.

½ cup chopped almonds

3 cups chopped green cabbage

2 cups chopped red cabbage

1 large organic apple, cored and grated (any apple variety will do)

3 large carrots, grated

½ cup crushed pineapple, drained

1–2 small green onions, chopped (optional)

Dressing

⅛ cup grapeseed or canola oil

⅛ cup apple cider vinegar (Bragg's is very good)

1–2 tablespoons agave nectar

1 tablespoon sesame seeds

Freshly ground pepper and salt

■ Combine the almonds, cabbage, grated apple, carrots, pineapple, and green onions in a large bowl. In a separate bowl, combine all of the dressing ingredients and whisk until well blended. Pour this mixture over the salad and toss to mix together well. Add salt and pepper to taste, and refrigerate until chilled.

VEGETABLE AND SIDE DISHES

BAKED DELICATA SQUASH

BLACK BEANS

CABBAGE AND GINGER SAUTÉ

GREEN BEANS WITH EDAMAME

GRILLED ASPARAGUS

HERBED BEETS AND ONION GRATIN

KALE WITH PEANUT SAUCE

LEEK SAUTÉ

MASHED SWEET POTATOES

MUSHROOM SAUTÉ

NOT-FRIED POTATOES

POLENTA

POTATO AND PEA CURRY

ROASTED BEETS

ROASTED POTATOES WITH HERBS

ROASTED RED BELL PEPPERS

ROASTED VEGETABLES

SALT AND PEPPER EDAMAME

SAUTÉED SPINACH WITH PINE NUTS

SLAVONIAN-STYLE GREEN BEANS

SPINACH DAL

SPINACH TOFU WITH PEANUT SAUCE

STUFFED BUTTERNUT SQUASH

STUFFED PORTOBELLO MUSHROOMS

VEGETABLE FRITTERS

VEGETABLE STIR-FRY

BAKED DELICATA SQUASH

SERVES 4

This simple and easy recipe can be made with several different kinds of squashes. Try this one, then try butternut, or acorn, and others; there are a lot to choose from.

2 large delicata squash, cut in half and seeded

2 tablespoons olive oil

Pinch of fresh rosemary or sage

Juice of 1 large orange

Freshly ground pepper

Coarse kosher salt

■ Preheat the oven to 350°F. Place the squash in a baking dish with sides, such as a jelly-roll pan, cut sides up. Brush the cut sides with the olive oil. Crush the rosemary over the cut sides and then pour the orange juice on top. Sprinkle with freshly ground pepper and coarse kosher salt, and bake for 40 to 50 minutes (pour a little water in the bottom of the pan during the baking process, to keep the squash skins from drying out). Adjust seasonings and serve.

BLACK BEANS

This recipe can be served alongside rice and a salad, or used as a filling for tacos or tostadas. It also goes very well with cornbread (page 122).

- 1 tablespoon organic extra-virgin olive oil
- 1 medium-size red onion, chopped
- 1 small carrot, chopped finely (optional)
- 1 red or green bell pepper, seeded and chopped
- ½ small jalapeño, chopped finely (optional)
- 3 cloves garlic, chopped
- 1 (15-ounce) can black beans, drained and rinsed
- 1 (14-ounce) can diced tomatoes
- 1½ teaspoons chile powder
- ¼ teaspoon cayenne
- 2 tablespoons chopped fresh cilantro
- ½–1 teaspoon sea salt or coarse kosher salt
- Freshly ground black pepper

■ Over medium heat, in a large skillet, heat the oil and sauté the onion for 2 to 3 minutes, or until it begins to become translucent. Add the chopped carrot, bell pepper, jalapeño, and garlic, and continue cooking for 8 to 10 minutes, or until the vegetables are fork tender. Add the black beans, tomatoes, chile powder, cayenne, and cilantro. Lower the heat to low and cook until the vegetables are completely cooked and the flavors have blended together, about 10 minutes more. Season to taste and serve hot.

CABBAGE AND GINGER SAUTÉ

SERVES 6

I love Savoy cabbage and blending it with ginger really makes for a good marriage of flavors. Of course, there are so many other cabbages that you could also use, such as bok choy, red or green cabbage, and Chinese (napa) cabbage; this would also work very well with Brussels sprouts, which are in the cabbage family.

1 tablespoon grapeseed oil

1 large Savoy cabbage, cored and chopped

1 tablespoon toasted sesame seed oil

1 teaspoon roasted red chile paste

1 tablespoon grated fresh ginger

Freshly ground pepper

Coarse kosher salt

■ Heat a large skillet or wok over medium-high heat and pour in the grapeseed oil. Add the cabbage and sauté for 2 to 3 minutes. Add the sesame oil, red chile paste, and ginger, and continue to sauté for another 2 to 3 minutes, until the cabbage is soft but not mushy. Season to taste with pepper and salt.

Note: If you don't have toasted sesame oil, regular sesame oil will work fine.

GREEN BEANS WITH EDAMAME

SERVES 4

Edamame (soybeans) are a great source of protein. If you have a soy allergy, you will not want to make this recipe—or just leave out the edamame and replace with fresh peas.

- 4 cups, ends trimmed, broken into bite-size lengths, fresh green beans
- 1 tablespoon olive oil
- 1 cup chopped red onion
- 1 cup shelled edamame
- 1 tablespoon finely chopped fresh ginger
- 4–5 cloves garlic, chopped
- 1 tablespoon wheat-free tamari sauce
- ¼ teaspoon sesame oil
- ¼ cup toasted walnuts (optional)
- ½ teaspoon sea salt or kosher salt
- ½ teaspoon freshly cracked pepper, or to taste

■ Steam the beans until they are crisp-tender, 6 to 7 minutes. Do not overcook. Remove from the steamer and set aside. In a large skillet, heat the olive oil over medium-high heat and add the onions. Sauté for 2 to 3 minutes, then add the edamame and continue cooking for 2 more minutes. Add the green beans, ginger, and garlic, and cook for 3 to 5 minutes. Add the tamari sauce, sesame oil, walnuts, and salt and pepper. Cook until beans are tender and adjust seasonings.

> Note: Edamame comes either in or out of the shell. For this recipe you want the ones without the shell.

GRILLED ASPARAGUS

You will need *skewers for this recipe if you plan to cook the asparagus outside on a barbecue grill. If you are cooking them indoors, use a ridged skillet.*

1½ pounds asparagus (about 2 bunches), trimmed but left whole
1–2 tablespoons olive oil
Coarse kosher salt
Freshly ground pepper

■ Heat your grill; if you are using bamboo skewers, soak them in water for 20 minutes before proceeding with the recipe. Skewer the asparagus sideways, about four stalks per skewer, so you can lay them on the grill easier and they won't fall through the grates. Prepare all of the asparagus this way, then lightly brush with the olive oil and sprinkle with kosher salt. Grill for 3 to 4 minutes per side.

HERBED BEETS AND ONION GRATIN

I could have named this recipe after Bruce again. When I dropped off samples of this dish at his market, he didn't show much interest, but the next day, when I stopped in to see what he thought about this recipe, he asked for more. Try it—if you like beets, you'll like this recipe.

5–6 roasted beets (page 69)

1 large onion, sliced

3 teaspoons organic olive oil

3 cloves garlic, chopped

½ cup chopped walnuts

6 tablespoons red or white wine

1 teaspoon dried tarragon

1 teaspoon chopped fresh parsley

■ Roast the beets as indicated on page 69 and, when cooled, cut into ½-inch slices. Sauté the onion in a skillet with 2 teaspoons of the olive oil until soft, then add the garlic and walnuts. Continue to sauté for 2 to 3 minutes, then add the wine and tarragon. Cook until the onions are tender.

■ Preheat the oven to 325°F. Pour the remaining teaspoon of olive oil into an 8- or 9-inch square baking dish and layer the beets inside. Spread the sautéed onion mixture on top of the beets, and sprinkle with the fresh parsley. Cover with foil and bake for 30 to 35 minutes.

KALE WITH PEANUT SAUCE

SERVES 4

Here is a wonderful recipe using peanut sauce. I really like the flavors, and kale is so good for us. I try to eat it at least once per week. Getting enough greens really is important in following a healthy diet.

1 large shallot or small onion, chopped

1 tablespoon olive oil

8 cups chopped kale

¼ cup Peanut Sauce (recipe follows)

Sea salt

Freshly ground pepper

Peanut Sauce

¼ cup organic peanut butter

¼ cup hot water

⅛ cup organic brown rice vinegar

1 tablespoon wheat-free tamari sauce

½ tablespoon agave nectar

½ tablespoon molasses

½ tablespoon chopped fresh cilantro

Pinch of red pepper flakes

■ In a large skillet, sauté the shallot in the olive oil over medium-high heat until soft, 3 to 4 minutes. Add the kale and continue to cook until crisp-tender, about 15 minutes. Meanwhile, whisk together all the sauce ingredients in a bowl.

■ Pour the peanut sauce over the kale mixture and heat through. Season to taste with salt and pepper.

> **Note: If you have an allergy to peanuts, you can make this recipe using cashew butter instead of peanut butter.**

LEEK SAUTÉ

One thing that is very important when cooking with leeks is the cleaning of them. You want to be sure to cut off the green part of the leeks and then run them through water over and over, to remove any dirt that is sticking between the layers. Leeks have a very subtle flavor and I use them often. If you don't have any leeks, don't despair; just use onions.

1 tablespoon olive oil

2 large leeks, well washed and chopped, white part only

2 medium-size shallots, chopped

4 cups cleaned and sliced mushrooms,

¼ cup red wine

¼ teaspoon fresh rosemary

½ teaspoon fresh thyme

½ teaspoon coarse kosher salt

Freshly ground pepper

■ Heat a large skillet over medium-high heat and pour in the oil. When it is hot, add the leeks and shallots, and sauté until soft, 3 to 4 minutes. Add the mushrooms, and continue to cook for another 8 to 10 minutes. Add the red wine and herbs, and simmer for 3 to 4 minutes. Lower the heat, simmer for a few minutes, and season to taste with salt and pepper. Serve over polenta or rice, if desired, or just serve as a side dish.

MASHED SWEET POTATOES

I have recently discovered maple butter. It is pure maple syrup—and unbelievably good! You can buy maple butter from your local health food store. The brand I use is Shady Maple Farms. Their ingredients are organic maple syrup and invert maple syrup. Consider substituting the maple butter for the margarine in this recipe. It's delicious. If you prefer creamier mashed potatoes, use hemp or soy milk in place of the orange juice.

2 pounds sweet potatoes or yams (I prefer yams), peeled and cubed

Juice of 2 oranges

¼ teaspoon freshly grated nutmeg

1 tablespoon vegan margarine (optional)

Coarse kosher salt

Freshly ground pepper

■ Cook the sweet potatoes in boiling water (or steam) until soft, 20 to 25 minutes. Drain, then mash the potatoes with the orange juice. Stir in the nutmeg, margarine, and salt and pepper to taste.

MUSHROOM SAUTÉ

I am a huge mushroom fan, although I don't eat them raw. I also love the flavors of wine and shallots mixed with mushrooms, so this is one recipe I think you will make over and over again. You may want to double it so you will have some left over. It's perfect to put on top of a baked potato or yam.

1 tablespoon olive oil

2 medium-size shallots, chopped

4 cups, cleaned, stemmed, and cut in half, cremini mushrooms (or any variety you like)

¼ cup Marsala cooking wine

1 tablespoon chopped fresh parsley

¼ teaspoon coarse kosher salt

Freshly ground pepper

■ In a large skillet, heat the olive oil over medium-high heat. Add the shallots and sauté until soft, 3 to 4 minutes. Add the mushrooms and continue to cook 4 to 5 minutes. Add the Marsala and cook until liquid evaporates, 8 to 10 minutes. Add the parsley, season with salt and pepper, and serve.

NOT-FRIED POTATOES

SERVES 4

I love baked fries, and these are even better because they are potatoes and yams. Yams have more nutritional value than potatoes, but red potatoes are better than white ones. Any vegetable with color is better for you; that's why we need to eat all kinds of vegetables: green ones, red ones, yellow ones, and so on.

2 large yams, peeled and cut into French fry–style strips (4 to 5 cups)

Olive oil (for oiling pan)

3–4 small red potatoes, peeled and cut into French fry–style strips

Sea salt and freshly ground pepper

Rosemary or Italian seasoning (optional)

■ Preheat the oven to 400°F. Place the potatoes on a cookie sheet that has been lightly greased with olive oil. Sprinkle with freshly ground pepper and sea salt. You can also sprinkle with rosemary or Italian seasoning, if you like. Bake until toasty, 40 to 45 minutes. Be sure to stir the potatoes during the baking process to ensure that they brown evenly.

POLENTA

This is great *served by itself, or seasoned with herbs as a side dish. You can also sauté vegetables and serve over the top of the polenta or use this as the base for Vegetable Ratatouille (page 104).*

4 cups soy or hemp milk
3 cups coarse cornmeal
½–1 teaspoon sea salt
Freshly ground pepper

■ Heat the milk in a 2-quart saucepan and, when it begins to boil, slowly add the cornmeal. Bring back to a boil, then lower the heat to low and cook until thick, stirring often, about 20 minutes. Be sure to stir this mixture, as you don't want it to stick to the bottom of the pan. Lower heat to the lowest setting if it continues to stick. Or add a bit more milk, if you prefer.

POTATO AND PEA CURRY

Curry—it's always good and hearty, and warming, too. If you like spicy food, you will need to adjust the spices here a bit, as this is a mild curry.

2 tablespoons olive oil

1 cup chopped onion

6 large red potatoes, peeled and cubed

2 cloves garlic, chopped finely

½ teaspoon ground cardamom

½ teaspoon ground coriander

¼ teaspoon chile powder

½ teaspoon ground cumin

¼ teaspoon ground turmeric

½ teaspoon ground cinnamon

½ teaspoon salt

1 cup light coconut milk

1½ cups fresh or frozen peas

½ cup raw cashews (optional)

½ cup chopped fresh cilantro

Freshly ground pepper

■ Heat a large skillet over medium-high heat and pour in 1 tablespoon of the oil. When it heats up, add the chopped onions, and sauté until they begin to soften, 3 to 4 minutes. Add the other tablespoon of oil and the potatoes, and sauté for 5 to 10 minutes. Add the spices and salt, and stir to coat the potatoes well. Continue to cook for 1 to 2 minutes, add the coconut milk, peas, and cashews, and stir well. Lower the heat to medium-low and cover. Cook until the potatoes are fork tender, 40 to 45 minutes. Add the cilantro, season to taste with salt and pepper, and stir to blend.

ROASTED BEETS

I never liked beets when I was younger, but they are growing on me. I love them in salads, which I recommend you use these for if you don't eat them all for dinner. I also like them just by themselves. Season the beets with herbs during the summer, right from your garden, and in the winter, use some freshly cracked pepper and coarse sea salt. They are a wonderful vegetable. Herbed Beets and Onion Gratin (page 61) uses these beets as its base.

5–6 beets
Olive oil
Salt and pepper

■ Preheat the oven to 375°F. Begin by cleaning the beets and cutting off the tops (save the beet greens to use in other recipes). Cut off most of the pointed part at the base, leaving about 1 inch. Line a cookie sheet with aluminum foil and lay the beets, whole, on the foil. Drizzle olive oil over the beets, then fold the foil around them so they are totally enclosed in the foil. Bake until they are soft but not mushy, 1 to 1½ hours. Remove from the oven and let cool. When they are cooled, cut into slices, season to taste with salt and pepper, and serve.

ROASTED POTATOES WITH HERBS

SERVES 4

My son Rory makes a recipe like this. *He learned it from our dear friends, Mike and Steve Burkhart. This is not their recipe, but my version of it. There is nothing like new baby potatoes roasted with olive oil and garlic. Yummy!*

16 baby red potatoes, scrubbed

1–2 tablespoons olive oil

4–5 cloves garlic, peeled

1 tablespoon dried parsley, or ¼ cup chopped fresh

½ teaspoon dried tarragon

1 teaspoon coarse kosher salt

½ teaspoon freshly ground pepper, or more to taste

■ Preheat the oven to 400°F. Pierce each potato a few times with a fork. Pour the olive oil into the bottom of a 9-inch square baking pan and add the pierced potatoes. Sprinkle the dried herbs on top and season lightly with salt and pepper. Roast in the oven until the potatoes are fork tender, about 45 minutes. Turn the potatoes during the roasting process a few times so they brown all over. Remove from the heat, and adjust seasonings to taste.

ROASTED RED BELL PEPPERS

MAKES ABOUT 1 POUND (COOKED)

I call for roasted bell peppers quite often in this cookbook, so I thought I had better tell you how to roast them yourself. It's really quite easy.

2 pounds red bell peppers
(4–5 large)

- In preparation for roasting the peppers, you will need to turn your oven to high broil and move the oven rack up to the top shelf. Line a cookie sheet with aluminum foil.
- Cut the peppers in half and scoop out all of the seeds and white pithy matter. Place the peppers cut side down on the cookie sheet and press them flat. Broil until they are black, about 20 minutes.
- Remove them from the oven and let cool slightly, then seal them in a large zipper-top plastic bag. Let the peppers sit in the bag for 15 to 20 minutes. Remove them from the bag and peel off their skins. They are ready to use or store for future use. They will keep in an airtight container for several days.

ROASTED VEGETABLES

My son Rory loves this recipe. I have made this recipe with several other vegetables, but this is our favorite. I serve it during the holidays but it's good anytime of the year.

- 2 tablespoons organic extra-virgin olive oil
- 5–6 cloves garlic, peeled but left whole
- 1 large red or sweet yellow onion, peeled and quartered
- 1 large yam, peeled and quartered
- ½ pound mushrooms, cleaned and stemmed
- 2 large carrots, cut in half lengthwise, then in half crosswise
- 2 cups, peeled, seeded, and cut into chunks, butternut squash
- 1 large zucchini, ends cut off, sliced in half lengthwise, then in half crosswise
- ½ cup chopped fresh parsley
- 3–4 tablespoons chopped fresh basil
- 1 teaspoon dried tarragon
- ½–1 teaspoon coarse kosher salt
- ½ teaspoon freshly cracked pepper, or to taste

■ Preheat the oven to 375°F. Pour a small amount of the olive oil onto the bottom of a 9 × 11-inch baking dish, and then place the vegetables in the pan, tossing them gently to coat with the oil. Drizzle some more of the olive oil on top, then sprinkle with the herbs and salt and pepper. Stir to coat with the oil and herbs. Bake uncovered for about 40–45 minutes or until done, making sure to stir occasionally while they roast so that they are cooked through and evenly roasted. The veggies should be crispy on the outside, and tender on the inside.

SALT AND PEPPER EDAMAME

Edamame (soybeans) are a great snack food. If you have allergies to soy, don't make these, but if you can eat soy, have these in place of chips or other less-than-desirable snacks. They are super easy to make and can be stored in a zipper-top plastic bag and taken on trips, in the car, or to work for a midafternoon snack.

1 pound frozen edamame in the pod

½ teaspoon coarse sea salt

Freshly ground pepper or Sichuan peppercorns

Italian seasoning (optional)

- Boil the edamame with a dash of salt until soft, 4 to 5 minutes. Follow with a cooling bath, placing the edamame pods in a pot of cold water as soon as they are tender. Drain and dry.
- Place the edamame in a large bowl and toss with the salt and pepper.

You could also use Sichuan peppercorns with this recipe. To make: lightly toast them, then grind and toss with the sea salt.

SAUTÉED SPINACH WITH PINE NUTS

If you like spicy food, add some red pepper flakes or a dash of hot sauce. It will really open up those sinuses.

- 1–2 tablespoons organic olive oil
- 3 cloves garlic, chopped
- ¼ cup pine nuts
- 1 bunch spinach, washed and chopped (4–6 cups)
- ¼ teaspoon coarse kosher salt
- Freshly ground pepper

■ In a large skillet, heat the oil over medium-high heat and add the garlic. Once it has become aromatic, about 1 minute, add the pine nuts and continue to sauté for 2 to 3 minutes, until they begin to brown slightly. Add the chopped spinach and cook until it wilts, 3 to 5 minutes. Season to taste with salt and pepper.

SLAVONIAN-STYLE GREEN BEANS

SERVES 4

My mother's side of the family is from the Old Country. We grew up eating this dish, along with many others that I love. My version isn't exactly like my grandmother's because I refuse to use so much olive oil. It's really great my way, but the Slavonians use more oil!

1 pound fresh green beans, chopped into 1-inch pieces

1 large baking potato, peeled and quartered

2–4 tablespoons olive oil

1–2 cloves garlic, chopped

1 large shallot or ½ onion, chopped

1 tablespoon chopped fresh parsley (optional)

Salt and pepper

■ Steam the green beans and potato together until tender (or if you want to prepare this as the Slavonians do, boil the potato and green beans together in a covered saucepan). While the beans and potatoes are cooking, heat a small skillet over medium heat and sauté the garlic and shallot in a little oil until soft, 4 to 5 minutes.

■ Once the potatoes and beans are cooked, remove them from the heat, drain, and coarsely mash them together. Add the garlic and shallots, and drizzle on more olive oil. Toss to coat. Season to taste with parsley, sea salt, and lots of pepper. You might want to add a bit more oil. (I wouldn't, but if I am really sharing this according to my family's instructions, then add more olive oil!)

SPINACH DAL

I used a bit too much mustard seed the first time I made this, and boy, did I hear about it. So, this is a scaled-back version. If you don't like mustard seeds, leave them out. It will not make a huge difference anyway. They add a unique flavor but aren't crucial to the recipe.

1 cup rinsed and picked over (to remove any debris) red or yellow lentils

1 tablespoon olive oil

1 medium-size onion, chopped

2 cloves garlic, chopped finely

1 tablespoon chopped fresh ginger

1 green chile, (about 2 tablespoons canned)

4 cups washed and chopped spinach (stems removed)

Pinch of mustard seeds (optional)

½ teaspoon cumin seeds

½ teaspoon ground turmeric

¼ cup chopped fresh cilantro

Salt

Freshly ground pepper

- In a 2-quart stockpot, place the lentils in 2 cups of water and cook until done, 40 to 45 minutes.
- In the meantime, heat a large skillet over medium heat and sauté the onions in the olive oil until soft, 4 to 5 minutes. Add the garlic, ginger, green chile, and spinach. Cook until the spinach is wilted, 4 to 5 minutes.
- When the lentils are cooked, add them to the vegetable mixture along with the herbs and spices. Mix well. Season with salt and pepper, as desired. Heat through and serve.

> Note: These can be served with the Dosas found on page 125.

SPINACH TOFU WITH PEANUT SAUCE

I love peanut sauce. It's one of my favorite things, so I had to make some recipes that called for it, so I could eat it. You can certainly use other leafy vegetables, such as kale or cabbage, in this recipe, but I prefer the combination of spinach and peanut butter.

Peanut Sauce

½ cup organic peanut butter

½ cup hot water

¼ cup organic brown rice vinegar

2 tablespoons wheat-free tamari sauce

1 tablespoon agave nectar

1 tablespoon molasses

1 tablespoon chopped fresh cilantro

Pinch of red pepper flakes

Spinach Tofu

2 tablespoons olive or grape-seed oil

1½ cups chopped onion

1 (12.3-ounce package) extra-firm silken tofu

4 cloves garlic, chopped finely

1 tablespoon finely chopped fresh ginger

1 bunch spinach, washed and chopped (4–6 cups)

Freshly ground pepper

Sea salt

Wheat-free tamari sauce (optional)

½ (16-ounce) package rice noodles, cooked (prepare according to package directions)

- Mix together the sauce ingredients in a medium-size bowl and set aside.
- In a large skillet, heat the oil and sauté the onion until soft, 3 to 4 minutes. Add the tofu and continue to cook for 2 to 3 minutes. Add the garlic and ginger, and cook for 1 to 2 minutes. Add the spinach and cook until it is wilted. Add the peanut sauce and heat through. Season with sea salt and lots of pepper. Add tamari sauce or other seasonings to taste. Serve over the cooked noodles.

STUFFED BUTTERNUT SQUASH

I make this recipe all the time. *I love the versatility of it. I can use up all my vegetables in one recipe, and it is filling and delicious. Sometimes I make it without the rice, instead adding quinoa, or I leave out the capers and eggplant, and add asparagus. It's really good, no matter what vegetables you use—as long as you stick to the herbs and spices, that's the secret: the flavor!*

1 large butternut squash (about 2 pounds)

1 tablespoon olive oil

1 large, well-washed leek or onion, chopped

⅓ cup chopped carrot

1 small zucchini, chopped

½ cup halved cleaned, stemmed mushrooms

½ cup chopped fresh or roasted red bell peppers

¼ cup chopped sun-dried tomatoes

⅓ cup chopped walnuts or (whole) pine nuts

3 cloves garlic, chopped finely

8–9 kalamata olives, pitted and cut in half

1–2 tablespoons capers (optional)

¼ cup cooked rice (optional)

¼ cup red or white wine

¼ cup chopped fresh parsley

1–2 tablespoons chopped fresh basil, or 1 teaspoon dried

¼–½ teaspoon coarse kosher salt

Freshly ground pepper

■ Preheat the oven to 400°F. Cut the ends off the squash and slice in half lengthwise. Scoop out and discard the seeds, then prick the squash all over with a fork (outside, not inside of squash). Drizzle a little olive oil on the cut side of the squash and place cut side down on a jelly-roll pan or any large baking dish with low sides. Pour a little water into the bottom of the pan. Roast until tender, 35 to 45 minutes.

■ In the meantime, heat a large skillet over medium-high heat and pour in the olive oil. When it is hot, add the chopped leek and sauté for a few minutes, until soft. Add the chopped/sliced carrot, zucchini, mushrooms, and bell peppers, and continue to sauté for 4 to 5 minutes. Add the sun-dried tomatoes, walnuts, and garlic, and continue to cook 1 to 2 minutes. Add the olives, capers, rice, and wine, and simmer for 3 to 4 minutes.

■ When the squash is soft, remove from the oven and let cool. Make lengthwise slit (not all the way through the skin) down the cut side center of each half and scoop out the squash along this center slit, making a groove for the sautéed vegetables. Cut the removed squash into bite-size chunks and add to the vegetable mixture. Stir in the parsley and basil, and add pepper and salt to taste. Stuff this mixture into both halves of the squash and place back on the baking sheet. Lower the oven temperature to 350°F and bake for about 30 minutes, or until heated through.

STUFFED PORTOBELLO MUSHROOMS

SERVES 4

These are really easy to make and have a great flavor. If you use vegan Parmesan cheese (note: most brands contain soy), you can sprinkle a little on top before you bake these, but I really don't think you need it. Everyone who tried these said they were just right exactly how they are. Each serving is one stuffed mushroom cap.

- 4 large portobello mushroom caps
- 1 tablespoon olive oil
- 1 cup chopped onion
- 1 small red bell pepper, seeded and chopped
- ¼ cup chopped yellow sweet pepper
- ½ cup finely chopped zucchini
- 2 cloves garlic, chopped
- 2 tablespoons chopped sun-dried tomatoes,
- 6 kalamata olives, pitted and chopped
- ¾ cup seeded and chopped fresh tomatoes
- 2 tablespoons pine nuts
- ½ teaspoon Italian seasoning
- 1 tablespoon chopped fresh basil,
- ½ teaspoon coarse kosher salt
- ¼ teaspoon freshly ground pepper, or to taste

- Preheat your oven's broiler. Clean the mushroom caps and remove the featherlike substance on the underside as well as the stem in the middle of the cap. Do this carefully, so you don't break the mushrooms. Lightly coat the mushrooms with olive oil, then place them on a cookie sheet and broil on both sides, 2 to 3 minutes on each side, or until they are soft. Remove from the oven and set aside. Turn off the broiler and preheat the oven to 350°F.

- In a large skillet, sauté the onion in the olive oil over medium heat until soft, 3 to 4 minutes. Add the peppers, zucchini, garlic, and sundried tomatoes, and continue to sauté until vegetables are tender. Add the olives, fresh tomatoes, and pine nuts, and continue to cook, stirring often, for 3 to 4 minutes. Add the Italian seasonings, basil, salt, and pepper.

- Carefully stuff this mixture into each mushroom cap, dividing the vegetables evenly among them, and bake for 15 minutes. Remove from the oven and serve.

VEGETABLE FRITTERS

These are very good. They remind me of an Indian dish I once had; I think it must be the spices. Speaking of spices, these are very spicy, so if you are not one to eat very spicy food, please omit the cayenne. To me, they are perfect as they are, but you might wish to serve them with fresh salsa.

⅔ cup garbanzo bean flour

5 tablespoons water

¼ teaspoon ground cumin

¼ teaspoon cayenne (optional)

¼ teaspoon ground turmeric

2 tablespoons chopped fresh cilantro

½ cup peeled and grated yam

½ cup finely chopped onion

2 cloves garlic, chopped

1–3 tablespoons grapeseed or canola oil

½ teaspoon baking soda

½ teaspoon salt

¼ teaspoon freshly ground pepper (or to taste)

■ In a large bowl, combine the garbanzo bean flour, water, cumin, cayenne, turmeric, and cilantro; with your hands, mix together until very well blended. Add the yam, onion, and garlic, and mix well.

■ Heat a large skillet over medium-high heat (closer to high than to medium) and pour in 1 to 2 tablespoons of the oil. When it is hot, scoop about 2 tablespoons of the mixture into your hands and form a ball. Carefully place the ball into the skillet and flatten it to form a patty. Add more balls and flatten them, until the skillet is full. Fry on each side until they are crispy, 6 to 8 minutes, then carefully flip over and fry on the other side. Remove from the skillet with a slotted spatula and place on a platter. Repeat with any remaining mixture. Season to taste with salt and pepper.

VEGETABLE STIR-FRY

This can be served over polenta, rice, or noodles (I serve it over brown rice). This is a very good stir-fry, but you can add whatever else you have in your refrigerator. I eat a lot of veggies and this combination is my favorite.

- 2 tablespoons olive oil
- 1 large onion, chopped
- 3 cups chopped broccoli
- 2 cups sliced carrots
- 1 cup chopped kale
- 2 cups chopped Savoy cabbage
- 2 cups cleaned, stemmed, and sliced mushrooms
- 1 red bell pepper, seeded and chopped
- 4–5 cloves garlic, chopped
- 1 teaspoon red curry paste
- 1–2 teaspoons wheat-free tamari sauce
- ¼–½ teaspoon coarse kosher salt
- ¼–½ teaspoon freshly cracked pepper

■ Heat a wok or large skillet over medium-high heat and pour in the oil. When it is hot, add the onion and sauté until the onion begins to soften, 3 to 4 minutes. Add the broccoli, carrots, and kale, and continue to sauté for 2 to 3 minutes. Add the cabbage, mushrooms, and red bell pepper, and continue to sauté. Add the garlic and sauté for 1 minute. Add the red curry paste and tamari sauce, and sauté until the veggies are crisp-tender. Season with salt and pepper, and serve.

MAIN DISHES

ANTIOXIDANT CHILI

ANTIOXIDANT RISOTTO

ASPARAGUS RISOTTO

CURRIED COCONUT AND SQUASH STEW

EGGPLANT ROLL-UPS

ITALIAN RISOTTO

ITALIAN-STYLE PASTA

J&J'S FAVORITE YAM AND BLACK BEAN BURRITOS

LENTIL STEW

LETTUCE WRAPS

MUSHROOM AND OLIVE PIZZA

NANCY'S FAVORITE MUSHROOM NUT LOAF

NO-MEAT MEATBALLS

PAD THAI

SPAGHETTI SQUASH WITH VEGETABLE RAGOUT

SPICY QUINOA PILAF

SPRING CASSEROLE

SPRING ROLLS

TOFU CHILI

VEGETABLE PAELLA

VEGETABLE RATATOUILLE OVER RICE

VEGGIE BURGERS

VEGGIE-STUFFED BELL PEPPERS

YAM ENCHILADAS WITH POMEGRANATE SAUCE

ANTIOXIDANT CHILI

I developed this recipe in late fall, when flu season started kicking up. I was teaching a cooking class, and I thought this would be a good recipe for the coming months. The class was happy because they got to take home samples.

1 tablespoon olive oil

1 large red onion, chopped

2 medium-size carrots, chopped

1 cup seeded and chopped green or red bell pepper

1 pound extra-firm silken tofu, drained and coarsely chopped

1 jalapeño, seeded and chopped

4 cloves garlic, chopped finely

1 (28-ounce) can organic tomatoes, diced

2 (15-ounce) cans beans (1 each black and red kidney, or any combination that you prefer), drained and rinsed

1 teaspoon ground cumin

1 tablespoon chile powder

¼ teaspoon red pepper flakes, or to taste

½ teaspoon sea salt or coarse kosher salt

Freshly ground pepper

Cornbread (page 122) (optional)

Guacamole (page 23) (optional)

■ Heat a large Dutch oven or skillet over medium heat. Pour in the olive oil and, when it heats up, add the onion and carrots, and sauté until the onion begins to soften, 4 to 5 minutes. Add the bell pepper, tofu, and jalapeño, and continue to sauté for another 5 minutes. Add the garlic and cook for 1 minute. Add the tomatoes, beans, cumin, chile powder, red pepper flakes, salt, and pepper, and cook until the flavors are blended, about 45 minutes. Serve with cornbread or top with guacamole.

ANTIOXIDANT RISOTTO

SERVES 4 TO 6

This is a very hearty main dish. If you wish, you could top it with vegan Parmesan cheese, but it really doesn't need it. I think you will enjoy it just the way it is. The secret to a good risotto is patience. It takes time to complete, about 45 minutes in all, but you will be very happy you put the time and energy into it when you sit down to enjoy it.

1 red onion, chopped

1½ tablespoons organic extra-virgin olive oil

2 cups chopped broccoli

1 cup peeled, seeded, and diced butternut squash

1 cup cleaned and halved mushrooms

2 cups washed and chopped spinach

3 cloves garlic, chopped

1 teaspoon chopped fresh ginger

½ cup pine nuts

¼ cup fresh chopped parsley

1 tablespoon chopped fresh tarragon

¼ cup white or red wine

1 (32-ounce) carton organic vegetable stock, or 4 cups homemade (page 34)

¾ cup uncooked Arborio rice

½ teaspoon sea salt or coarse kosher salt

½ teaspoon freshly ground pepper, or to taste

■ In a large Dutch oven or skillet, sauté the onion in 1 tablespoon of the olive oil for 2 minutes over medium-high heat, then add the broccoli and butternut squash and continue to cook, until the veggies are beginning to cook through but are not mushy. (Add more oil if needed, so the vegetables do not stick to the skillet.) Add the mushrooms, spinach, garlic, and ginger at this point, and continue cooking for 5 minutes or so. Add the pine nuts, herbs, and wine, and sauté until most of the wine is absorbed. Remove from the heat and set this mixture aside.

■ In a 3- to 4-quart saucepan, heat the vegetable stock to boiling. This needs to be kept hot while you prepare the rice.

■ Heat a second large Dutch oven over medium-high heat. Pour in a small amount of olive oil (maybe 1 teaspoon) and add the rice. Stir it around so that the rice is coated with the oil and, when it begins to brown lightly, start to add the hot vegetable stock, one ladleful at a time. Each time you add the stock, let the rice absorb the stock completely before you add another ladleful. Keep stirring the mixture as it cooks. This process will take some time, about 30 minutes in all. After you have added all of the vegetable stock, and the rice is cooked, stir the cooked vegetables into the rice and season with salt and pepper. Heat through and serve.

ASPARAGUS RISOTTO

SERVES 4

Risotto takes time, but in the end it is worth it. Winter is a great time for risotto, but so is spring when asparagus is young and tender.

1 tablespoon olive oil

2 large shallots, chopped finely (about ½ cup)

1 bunch asparagus, chopped (about 3 cups)

3 cloves garlic, chopped finely

2 cups cleaned and sliced mushrooms

1 teaspoon chopped fresh tarragon

1 tablespoon chopped fresh parsley

1 tablespoon basil

1 (32-ounce) carton organic vegetable stock, or 4 cups homemade (page 34)

1 cup uncooked Arborio rice

¼ cup white wine or water

¼ cup pine nuts

■ Place 1 tablespoon of the oil in a large Dutch oven or stockpot, and heat over medium-high heat. Add the shallots and asparagus, and sauté for 5 to 6 minutes. Add the garlic and continue to sauté, about 1 minute. Add the mushrooms and herbs, and cook until the mushrooms begin to soften, about 2-3 minutes. Once the vegetables are fork tender, remove from the pan and set aside.

■ In the meantime, heat the vegetable stock in a saucepan to boiling, and keep it hot. You are going to use the hot stock to add to the rice as it continues to cook. If you add the stock cool, it will add to the cooking time, so keep it simmering throughout the cooking process.

■ Add the last tablespoon of oil to the pan used for the vegetables and heat again over medium-high heat. Add the rice and stir until it begins to brown lightly. Begin to add the stock one ladleful at a time, allowing the rice to absorb the broth completely before adding another ladle of stock. Add the wine and continue this process (it takes at least 30-35 minutes) until all of the broth has been added and the rice is cooked through. Add the vegetables and pine nuts to the rice once it is cooked, and heat through. Serve hot.

CURRIED COCONUT
AND SQUASH STEW

I am a fan of coconut milk, and I also love squash, so why not combine the two? It's not too spicy but just right. You will notice the ingredients list specifies two tablespoons of olive oil but I only mention using one. If you can get away with just one, then go with it. If the vegetables start to stick when you are sautéing them, add the other tablespoon.

2 tablespoons olive oil

1 cup finely chopped red onion

1 teaspoon diced fresh ginger

1 large red bell pepper, seeded and chopped

1 pound extra firm silken tofu, cubed

3 cloves garlic, chopped finely

1½ cups peeled, seeded, and cubed butternut, or delicata squash

1 tablespoon seeded and finely chopped jalapeño

2 teaspoons mild curry powder

1 cup hemp or soy milk

1 cup light coconut milk

1 tablespoon fresh lime juice

¼–½ cup chopped fresh cilantro

½ teaspoon coarse kosher salt

Freshly ground pepper

■ In a large Dutch oven or stockpot, heat 1 tablespoon of the olive oil over medium heat and sauté the onion until soft, 4 to 5 minutes. Add the ginger, bell pepper, tofu, garlic, squash, and jalapeño, and continue to sauté until the squash is fork tender, about 15 minutes. Add the curry powder and the hemp and coconut milks, and heat to a boil. Lower the heat to medium-low and cook until flavors are blended, about 5-10 minutes. Add the lime juice, cilantro, salt and pepper to taste, and serve.

> Note: To make your own curry, see page 68.
> Use the spices assembled for the curried peas
> and potatoes recipe.

EGGPLANT ROLL-UPS

I came up with this idea to use the leftovers from *Veggie-Stuffed Bell Peppers (page 106).* I have also made roll-ups from the ingredients in *Italian-Style Pasta (page 90).* This is a fun recipe, because you just grill the strips, fill them with whatever you want, roll them up, cover them with the sauce, and bake them in the oven. Dinner is served!

1½ cups prepared filling for Veggie-Stuffed Bell Peppers (page 106)

1 large eggplant, peeled and sliced thinly lengthwise

1 (15-ounce) can organic tomato sauce

1 tablespoon chopped fresh basil

1 teaspoon dried oregano

1 tablespoon chopped fresh parsley

¼ cup red or white wine

¼ teaspoon sea salt

Fresh cracked pepper

- After you prepare the filling, do the following:
- Preheat the oven to 350°F.
- Grill the eggplant slices to soften them up. If you don't have a grill, sauté them just until they soften, as you want them to be able to roll up.
- In a bowl, mix together the tomato sauce, herbs, wine, and salt and let the mixture sit for a few minutes so the flavors blend together. Pour half of this mixture into a baking dish. Place about ⅛ cup of the filling in the middle of each slice of eggplant and roll up. Place the rolls on top of the sauce in the pan. After all the eggplant rolls are assembled, spoon the rest of the sauce over them and sprinkle with pepper. Bake until the sauce is bubbly and the eggplant rolls are soft, about 30 minutes.

> **Note:** You can use a George Foreman Grill to prepare the eggplant instead of sautéing, if you prefer.

ITALIAN RISOTTO

This is great as a main dish with salad on the side. I mentioned earlier, the secret to making risotto is having the patience and time to prepare it. It does take almost an hour to make this dish, as you need to cook the rice slowly, a ladleful at a time.

2 tablespoons olive oil

1 small onion, chopped

2 cups peeled, seeded, and cubed butternut or other winter squash

2 cups washed and chopped spinach

1 large zucchini, chopped

3–4 cloves garlic, minced

⅓ cup preferably fresh peas

½ cup sliced cremini mushrooms

1 cup chopped walnuts

¼ cup red wine

¼ cup chopped roasted red bell pepper (page 71)

10 kalamata olives, pitted and cut in half

2 tablespoons chopped fresh basil

1 teaspoon dried oregano

¾ cup uncooked Arborio rice

1½ (32-ounce) cartons organic vegetable stock, or 6 cups homemade (page 34)

½ cup chopped fresh parsley

¼ teaspoon sea salt

Freshly ground pepper (at least ¼ teaspoon or more!)

■ In a Dutch oven or large, deep skillet, heat 1 tablespoon of the olive oil and add the onion. Sauté over medium-high heat until the onion begins to soften, 3 to 4 minutes. Add the butternut squash, and continue to cook about 5 to 8 minutes, or until squash is fork tender. Add the spinach, zucchini, garlic, peas, and mushrooms, and continue to cook for 3 to 4 minutes. Add the walnuts, wine, roasted red bell peppers, olives, basil, and oregano. Remove from the skillet and set aside.

■ Meanwhile, in a 2 quart saucepan, heat the vegetable stock to boiling, and keep it hot.

■ Heat 1 tablespoon of oil in a Dutch oven over medium-high heat. When the oil is hot, add the rice and stir to coat with the oil.

■ Once the rice begins to pop or brown slightly, begin adding the hot vegetable stock into the Dutch oven. Cook the rice until all of the stock is absorbed, then add another ladleful of stock. Continue this process until the rice is cooked and all of the stock has been added. Once this is complete, add the vegetables to the rice and mix well. Add the parsley, fresh ground pepper, and salt to taste. Heat through.

ITALIAN-STYLE PASTA

SERVES 6

This is another *favorite recipe for many of my taste testers. It's so full of flavor and the kalamata olives really give it some zip. I just love the combination of vegetables and pasta.*

1 tablespoon olive oil

1 large onion, chopped

¼ cup chopped roasted red bell pepper

¼ cup chopped sun-dried tomatoes

5–6 cloves garlic, chopped

1 cup washed and chopped spinach

¼ cup red wine

½ cup artichoke hearts in oil, or eggplant, peeled and cubed

1 cup seeded and diced fresh tomatoes

3 tablespoons chopped fresh basil

1 tablespoon chopped fresh parsley

1 teaspoon Italian seasoning

¼–½ cup pine nuts

¼ cup capers (optional)

20 kalamata olives, pitted and cut in half

8–12 ounces uncooked rice penne, prepared according to package directions

■ Pour the oil into a Dutch oven or large sauté pan, and heat over medium-high heat. Add the onion and sauté until soft, 4 to 5 minutes. Add the roasted red bell pepper, sun-dried tomatoes, and garlic. Continue to cook for 2 to 3 minutes. Add the spinach and cook for another 2 to 3 minutes. Add the wine, artichoke hearts, fresh tomatoes, herbs, pine nuts, capers, and olives. Lower the heat to low and simmer this mixture until it is heated through and the vegetables are tender. Season to taste with salt and pepper. Pour the sauce over the cooked penne and toss. It is magnifico!

J&J'S FAVORITE YAM
AND BLACK BEAN BURRITOS

SERVES 4 TO 6

Jeffrey and Jessie loved this recipe. I made it when I went to visit them in California, and they begged for the recipe before I left. Since I had just intended to have them taste-test the recipe, I was thrilled that they gave it the thumbs-up by asking for it. I think you'll find that this is so filling that you don't need to serve it with a tortilla but, boy, can you make a *mean* burrito with this filling! Top it off with guacamole, and you are in heaven!

2 large yams

1 tablespoon olive oil

1 cup chopped onion

2 tablespoons seeded and chopped red bell pepper (roasted is great, but not necessary)

1 small jalapeño, diced

2 cloves garlic, chopped

1 cup seeded and diced tomato

1 cup tomato salsa

1 teaspoon chile powder

1 teaspoon ground cumin

1 (15-ounce) can organic black beans, drained and rinsed

⅔ cup chopped fresh cilantro

2 tablespoons lime juice

½ teaspoon salt (coarse kosher is best)

¼–½ teaspoon freshly ground black pepper

8 rice or hemp tortillas

Guacamole (page 23) (optional)

- There are two ways you can prepare the yams for this recipe: prick the yams all over with a fork, and bake in the oven at 400 degrees until soft but not mushy; or prick them with a fork and microwave until soft, 5 to 6 minutes on high (time depends on the size of the yams).

- While the yams bake, heat a large skillet over medium-high heat and sauté the onion in the olive oil until soft, 3 to 4 minutes. Add the red bell pepper and jalapeño, and continue sautéing for another 3 to 4 minutes, or until the pepper becomes soft. Add the garlic and cook for 1 minute. Peel the yams, cut into cubes, and add to the vegetable mixture. Add the diced tomatoes, salsa, spices, black beans, cilantro and lime juice. Heat through. Season with plenty of freshly ground pepper and coarse kosher sea salt.

- Heat the tortillas and fill with the mixture. Serve with guacamole if desired.

LENTIL STEW

Lentil stew is *so warming and this one is very hearty. It will fill you up and make you feel good.*

1 tablespoon olive oil

1 large onion, chopped

2 carrots, chopped

2 stalks celery, chopped

1 cup washed and chopped spinach

1 cup cooked and chopped green beans

1 (32-ounce) carton organic vegetable stock, or 4 cups homemade (page 34)

1 bay leaf

1 cup red or green lentils, well rinsed and picked over (to remove any debris)

Pinch of red pepper flakes

1 teaspoon salt

½ teaspoon fresh grated pepper, or more to taste

■ In a Dutch oven or large kettle, heat the oil over medium-high heat and add the onions. Sauté until soft, 4 to 5 minutes. Add the carrots and celery, and continue to cook for 3 to 4 minutes. Add the spinach, cooked green beans, vegetable stock, bay leaf, lentils, and red pepper flakes. Lower the heat to medium-low and cook until the lentils are soft, about 20 minutes. Season with salt and pepper

LETTUCE WRAPS

Lettuce wraps are a wonderful way to make a quick and easy lunch. You can use all kinds of things to make a wrap. I have provided two options, Mexican and Greek style. At a restaurant I recently enjoyed a Caesar salad wrap, so you might consider that, too. Black beans would be great in a lettuce wrap with some guacamole or sliced avocado.

Mexican-Style Wrap

¼ cup J&J's Yam and Bean Burrito filling (page 91)

2 large romaine hearts or butter-leaf lettuce leaves, washed and patted dry

1–2 slices avocado, or a dollop of guacamole (page 23)

1 tablespoon salsa (page 26)

■ Heat the burrito mixture in a small skillet, then spoon it onto the lettuce leaves. Add the avocado and salsa, and roll up.

Greek-Style Wrap

1 tomato, seeded and chopped

½ cucumber, peeled and chopped

1 green onion or shallot, chopped

1 clove garlic, chopped

1–2 teaspoons olive oil

1 tablespoon lemon juice

Salt

Freshly ground pepper

A few kalamata olives, pitted and chopped

Chopped fresh herbs of choice (e.g., a pinch of oregano and some basil leaves)

Artichoke hearts, chopped red bell pepper, or chopped red onions (optional)

2 large romaine hearts or butter-leaf lettuce leaves, washed and patted dry

■ Combine the vegetables and garlic with the olive oil, lemon juice, and salt and pepper. Add the olives and herbs. Toss together and add anything else you can think of, such as artichoke hearts, red bell peppers, or red onions. Roll up the mixture in the lettuce leaves and you have a salad in a wrap! (You can also use the rice or hemp tortillas in place of the lettuce leaves.)

MUSHROOM AND OLIVE PIZZA

I have a friend who isn't too fond of "my style of food" so when she said she really liked this pizza, I knew I was headed in the right direction. Thank you, Maggie, for your willingness to give this pizza a try!

1 tablespoon olive oil

½ cup chopped shallots or onions

4 cloves garlic, chopped

2 cups cleaned and sliced mushrooms

⅓ cup kalamata olives, pitted and sliced in half

1–2 tablespoons pine nuts

2 tablespoons chopped fresh basil, 2 teaspoons dried

1 (6-ounce) can tomato puree

½ teaspoon coarse kosher salt

Freshly ground pepper

1 recipe pizza crust (page 130)

■ Preheat the oven to 350°F.

■ In a large skillet, heat the olive oil over medium-high heat. Add the shallots and sauté until soft. Add the garlic and mushrooms. Continue to sauté until the mushrooms are soft, 4 to 5 minutes. Add the olives, pine nuts, and basil. Add the tomato puree. Stir to mix well. Season to taste with salt and pepper.

■ Spread this mixture over the pizzacrust. Bake at 350°F for 15 minutes, then increase the oven temperature to 450°F degrees and bake for 10 minutes more. The pizza should be heated all the way through. Keep an eye on the pizza after you raise the heat, to be sure it does not burn. If it is too hot, reduce the heat and continue cooking until done (oven temperatures vary). Cool on a wire rack.

NANCY'S FAVORITE MUSHROOM NUT LOAF

SERVES 4

This is a very hearty meal. It certainly doesn't look like a typical "meat loaf" but boy is it good. Try putting the cashew gravy on top. You will love it!

1–2 tablespoons olive oil

1 cup chopped onion

2 cloves garlic, chopped finely

2 cups chopped cremini or other mushrooms

¾ cup chopped raw cashews

1 cup chopped walnuts

½ cup Marsala cooking wine

1 tablespoon arrowroot powder

Juice of 1 medium-size lemon

¼ cup sorghum flour

¼ teaspoon dried rosemary

½ teaspoon dried thyme

½ teaspoon sea salt or coarse kosher salt

Lots of freshly ground pepper

■ Preheat the oven to 350°F and have ready a 9 × 5 × 3-inch loaf pan.

■ Heat a large skillet over medium-high heat and pour in 1 tablespoon of the oil. When it is hot, add the onion and sauté until it begins to soften, 5 to 6 minutes. Add the garlic, mushrooms, and nuts, and continue to cook, stirring often. If the mixture begins to stick to the bottom of the skillet, then add a little more oil. Add the Marsala, arrowroot, lemon juice, sorghum flour, rosemary, and thyme. Continue to cook until the mixture begins to thicken, about 1 to 2 minutes. Season with salt and pepper and then press the mixture into the loaf pan.

■ Bake for about 30 minutes, or until browned on top. Serve in slices.

> **Note: You may wish to double the recipe so you will have leftovers!**

NO-MEAT MEATBALLS

SERVES 6

This recipe took a bit of work, but I finally found a combination that held together. You will love the flavor of these no-meat meatballs. They are really good just as they are, or delightful served with Cashew Gravy (page 172).

1 tablespoon olive oil, plus more for sautéing

¼ cup well-washed and chopped leeks, white part only

½ cup chopped red onion

3 cloves garlic, chopped

2 cups cleaned and finely diced mushrooms

1 cup cooked brown rice or rice medley (I cook the rice in vegetable stock to give it more flavor.)

½ cup cooked, mashed potatoes

½ cup chopped pecans or walnuts

¼ teaspoon dried rosemary

1 tablespoon fresh parsley

Pinch of dried thyme

1 tablespoon organic tomato paste

½ teaspoon coarse kosher salt or sea salt

¼ teaspoon freshly ground pepper, or more to taste

■ Preheat the oven to 350°F if you wish to bake rather than sauté the meatballs.

■ In a large skillet, heat the oil and sauté the leek and onion over medium-high heat for 4 to 5 minutes. Add the garlic and continue to cook for a minute or two. Add the mushrooms and cook until they are soft. Transfer the cooked vegetables to a large mixing bowl. Add the cooked rice, mashed potatoes, pecans, herbs, tomato paste, and salt and pepper.

■ Press tightly into balls (press hard, so they'll stay together) and sauté on all sides in a large skillet, in 1 to 2 tablespoons of olive oil over medium-high heat. Once the balls are browned, lower the heat to medium low and cook until heated through, about 5 minutes.

■ If you prefer to bake the meatballs, place them on a large cookie sheet and bake at 350°F until heated through, about 30 minutes.

> **Note: You could replace the mashed potatoes with mashed sweet potatoes or yams in this recipe, too.**

PAD THAI

This is one of my favorite dishes when dining out. I love Thai food, and since it's made with rice noodles, I can enjoy it without worrying about gluten. If you are allergic to peanuts, please leave them out, or substitute cashews. You can add any vegetables you like to Pad Thai. It will taste just as good.

- 1 tablespoon grapeseed oil
- 2 cups chopped onions
- ½ cup chopped carrots
- 12 ounces extra-firm silken tofu, cubed
- ¼ cup apple cider vinegar (such as Bragg's)
- ¼ cup wheat-free tamari sauce
- 2 tablespoons agave nectar
- 1 teaspoon red curry paste
- 1–2 tablespoons organic peanut butter
- 1 cup washed and drained bean sprouts
- 6 ounces uncooked rice noodles (rice sticks), prepared according to package directions
- 4 green onions, chopped
- 1 tablespoon lime juice

■ In a large skillet, heat the oil over medium-high heat and add the onions and carrots. Sauté until the onions become soft, 4 to 5 minutes. Add the tofu and continue to cook, stirring occasionally, for 4 to 5 minutes. Add the vinegar, tamari sauce, agave nectar, red curry paste, peanut butter, and bean sprouts. Toss to coat, and heat through.

■ Pour the tofu mixture over the noodles, and garnish with the green onions and lime juice.

SPAGHETTI SQUASH
WITH VEGETABLE RAGOUT

SERVES 6 TO 8

It is really quite remarkable how much spaghetti squash is like real noodles, only better. You want to be sure you roast it until it is soft. Often the squash will have baking directions stuck right on the side (remove these before baking!). Spaghetti squash is so versatile—you can top it with many things—but this is my favorite recipe for it.

1 spaghetti squash (about 2 pounds)

1 tablespoon olive oil

1 large onion, chopped

1 medium-size zucchini, chopped (about 1½ cups)

3 cups Swiss chard

½ cup chopped roasted red bell pepper (page 71)

4 ounces cremini mushrooms (about 8), chopped

4 cloves garlic, chopped

1 (14.5-ounce) can diced or whole tomatos

1 tablespoon capers

2 tablespoons chopped fresh basil, or more if desired

⅛ cup red wine

¼ teaspoon freshly ground pepper, or to taste

½ teaspoon coarse kosher salt

- Preheat the oven to 400°F degrees and place the squash directly on the oven rack. Bake until soft, about 1 hour. Remove from the oven.

- While the squash is cooking, place a large skillet over medium-high heat and pour in the olive oil. Add the onion, zucchini, and Swiss chard, and sauté for 8 to 10 minutes. Add the roasted bell pepper, mushrooms, and garlic, and cook for 5 minutes. Add the diced tomatoes and capers, and continue to cook for 1 to 2 minutes. Add the basil and wine, and cook until the flavors blend, 2 to 3 minutes.

- Cut the squash in half. Using a large spoon or fork, scoop all of the "noodles" out and place in a large bowl. Add the vegetable mixture and toss to mix well. Season with pepper and salt, and serve immediately.

SPICY QUINOA PILAF

SERVES 4

Quinoa is such a versatile grain. I love its nutty flavor and that it is chock full of protein. It is easy to cook with and is a great noodle replacement in soups and stews. If this is too spicy for you, leave out the jalapeño.

- 1–2 tablespoon olive or grapeseed oil
- 1 small onion, chopped finely
- ½ small zucchini, chopped
- 2 teaspoons finely chopped jalapeño (optional)
- 1 teaspoon finely chopped fresh ginger
- 3 cups vegetable stock (storebought or homemade, page 34)
- ¼ teaspoon ground cardamom
- ½ teaspoon ground coriander
- ½ teaspoon ground cumin
- Pinch of cayenne
- 1½ cups uncooked quinoa, rinsed and drained
- 3 tablespoons chopped fresh cilantro
- ¼ cup toasted pine nuts (toast ahead of time in a small skillet over medium-high heat for a few minutes, until the nuts begin to brown)
- Sea salt
- Freshly ground pepper

■ Heat the oil in a large skillet and sauté the onion for 3 to 4 minutes. Add the zucchini, jalapeño, and ginger, and sauté for another 3 to 4 minutes. Add the vegetable stock and all the spices (except the cilantro) as well as the quinoa. Bring to a boil, then lower the heat and cover. Simmer until all the liquid is absorbed, 10 to 12 minutes. Add the cilantro and roasted pine nuts, and stir. Season to taste with salt and freshly ground pepper. Serve hot.

SPRING CASSEROLE

SERVES 4

This is a lovely dish. The flavors in this recipe really blend together nicely. I recommend you use a subtle milk substitute in this recipe, so it doesn't end up overpowering the flavors. I have used both soy and hemp, and they work fine.

2 cups halved baby carrots

1 tablespoon olive oil

1 large red onion, chopped

2 small shallots, chopped, or ¼ cup additional chopped onion

2 cloves garlic, chopped

½ pound asparagus, washed, ends trimmed, and cut into thirds

½ teaspoon saffron

4 cups washed and chopped spinach

1 cup fresh mushrooms, preferably chanterelles or cremini (less expensive)

1 cup organic fresh peas

1 teaspoon fresh thyme

½ cup white wine

1 cup mushroom or vegetable stock (store-bought or home-made, page 34)

1 cup soy, coconut, hemp, or half-coconut, half-other milk

½ teaspoon freshly ground pepper

¼ teaspoon sea salt or coarse kosher salt

- Preheat the oven to 350°F. Lightly spray a 9-inch square pan with vegetable oil nonstick spray.
- Steam the carrots until fork tender. In a large skillet or Dutch oven, heat the olive oil over medium high heat and add the onions and shallots. Sauté until they begin to soften, 5 to 6 minutes. Add the garlic, asparagus, saffron, spinach, carrots, mushrooms, peas, and thyme. Cook for 5 to 6 minutes, or until the spinach is wilted and the asparagus is fork tender. Add the wine and cook until it is just about evaporated. Add the mushroom or vegetable stock and simmer until the mixture has reduced by about half. Add the soy/hemp milk, salt and pepper and bring to a simmer. Simmer for 2 to 3 minutes.
- Transfer the vegetable mixture to the prepared pan and bake until lightly browned and heated through, about 30 minutes.

SPRING ROLLS

SERVES 8

I like using rice wraps for spring rolls, but a hemp tortilla is a nice variation. If you prefer a more traditional spring roll, then use the commercial rice wrap. The great thing about spring rolls is that you can add various ingredients to them and they still taste good dipped in a peanut sauce.

3–4 ounces rice noodles, chopped into 1–2-inch pieces

1 cup julienned snow peas

1 large avocado, peeled and sliced very thinly

2 medium-size carrots, sliced thinly lengthwise

1 large cucumber, sliced lengthwise, thinly

½ cup chopped water chestnuts

8 hemp tortillas

Peanut sauce (page 176) or commercially prepared sweet-and-sour sauce (optional)

- There are two ways you can prepare the rice noodles. On the package, it tells you to soak them in warm water until soft but not mushy, which takes 30 to 45 minutes. I usually want quicker results, so I place the noodles in boiling water, cover the pot, then turn off the heat. After 10 minutes, I drain the noodles.
- Place the vegetables, avocado, and water chestnuts in a large bowl and toss them together. Add the cooled rice noodles and mix together.
- Hemp rolls taste great, but they don't roll up really easily without breaking, so I recommend that you soften them up by heating a large skillet and turning it up to a moderately high temperature. Add a small drip of oil, then a tortilla, and swirl it around until it softens up. Remove from the heat and place some of the vegetable mixture in the middle and roll it up. Continue this process until you have used all of the tortillas and mixture. Serve with peanut or sweet-and-sour sauce.

TOFU CHILI

SERVES 4 TO 6

This recipe is *great for potlucks or a Sunday ball game with friends. It is easy to make, fills you up, and tastes great. I like to make it on the weekend so I have an easy lunch throughout the week. I top it with guacamole and serve with chips, too.*

1 tablespoon olive oil

1 large onion, chopped

1 cup chopped green bell pepper

2 cloves garlic, chopped

2 large carrots, chopped

1 pound extra-firm silken tofu, or any other firm tofu, cubed

2 (15-ounce) cans beans (1 can each black and red kidney, or use whatever kind you prefer)

1 (28-ounce) can diced or crushed tomatoes

1 tablespoon chile powder

1 teaspoon ground cumin

¼ teaspoon red pepper flakes

Salt and pepper

Cornbread (page 122) (optional)

■ Sauté the onion, pepper, garlic, and carrots in the oil, in a deep skillet or Dutch oven, over medium-high heat. Once the onion becomes soft, 4 to 5 minutes, add the tofu and continue to sauté for 8 to 10 minutes. Add the beans, tomatoes, chile powder, cumin, and red pepper flakes. Bring this mixture to a boil, then lower the heat and cook for 30 to 40 minutes, until cooked through. Season to taste with salt and pepper. Serve with cornbread, if desired.

VEGETABLE PAELLA

SERVES 4

This is a one-pot dinner. There is every-thing here that you need. If you wish to serve it with a salad, that's wonderful, but you have tons of vegetables and healthy carbs in this paella.

1–2 tablespoons olive oil

1 large red onion, chopped finely

1 large leek, well washed and chopped (only the white part)

1 large red bell pepper, seeded and chopped

1 cup cleaned, stemmed, and halved mushrooms

4 cloves garlic, chopped finely

¼ teaspoon fennel seeds

1 cup brown basmati or other paella-style rice

3 cups vegetable stock (store-bought or homemade, page 34)

⅓ cup red wine

2 tablespoons chopped fresh parsley

½ teaspoon paprika

Pinch of saffron (optional)

¼ cup chopped fresh cilantro

½ teaspoon freshly ground pep-per, or to taste

½ teaspoon coarse kosher salt, or to taste

■ Heat the oil in a large skillet or Dutch oven over medium heat and sauté the onion and leek until soft, 4 to 5 minutes. Add the bell pepper, mushrooms, and garlic, and continue to cook for another 6 to 8 minutes. Add the fennel seeds, rice, vegetable stock, and wine, and bring to a boil. Then lower the heat to low and simmer until the liquid is absorbed, 15 to 18 minutes. Add the parsley, paprika, saffron, and cilantro, turn off the heat, and cover the pan. Let the rice mixture sit for 5 minutes. Add salt and pepper to taste.

VEGETABLE RATATOUILLE over RICE

SERVES 6

I made this recipe one night when my friend Dara was here. She just raved about it, and told me the name Vegetable Ratatouille over Rice didn't do the recipe justice. It is what it is, and you'd better try this one, 'cause it's a "keeper." As a change, serve over Polenta (page 67) instead of rice.

Rice

4 cups water

2 cups brown rice (I recommend Lundberg Family Farms brand)

Pinch of salt

Ratatouille

1 tablespoon olive oil

1 large onion, chopped

12 baby or 2 large carrots, chopped

2 cups peeled, cubed yams (cut into 1-inch cubes)

1 large red bell pepper, seeded and chopped (about 2 cups)

1 medium-size eggplant, peeled and cut into cubes (about 3 cups)

4 cloves garlic, chopped

12–15 cremini mushrooms, cut in half

2 small zucchinis, sliced

1 (28-ounce) can diced tomatoes

1 (15-ounce) can garbanzo beans (chickpeas), drained

½ cup vegetable stock (store-bought or homemade, page 34)

¼ cup chopped fresh basil, or 1 tablespoon dried

1 teaspoon Italian seasoning

¼ cup chopped fresh parsley

1 teaspoon sea salt or coarse kosher salt

Freshly ground pepper

- Prepare the rice: bring the water to a boil in a 2-quart saucepan and add the rice and salt. Lower the heat to medium-low, cover, and simmer until rice is cooked, about 50 minutes.

- While the rice cooks, prepare the ratatouille: In a large skillet, heat the olive oil over medium-high heat and add the onion. Sauté until it begins to soften, then add the carrots, yam, bell pepper, eggplant, and garlic. Continue to sauté, for 5 minutes. Add the mushrooms, zucchini, tomatoes, garbanzo beans, vegetable stock, and seasonings, and continue to cook for another 8 to 10 minutes, or until the vegetables are fork tender but not mushy. Season with salt and pepper, and adjust herbs, if desired.

- When the rice is done, remove the lid, fluff, and top with the ratatouille.

VEGGIE BURGERS

Boy, oh boy, did my taste tester Nancy love these. Nancy works with people who are always looking for a vegetarian/vegan/gluten-free burger that tastes good. She said, "Suzi, can you create a veggie burger?" I said I would try, and she reported back, "You did it!" So, if you are hungry for a burger, this is worth trying. I like these served with guacamole (page 23) or salsa (page 26).

1 cup frozen roasted corn (Trader Joe's carries this)

½ cup finely chopped red onion

2 cloves garlic, chopped finely

¼ cup seeded and chopped red bell pepper

1 cup cooked long-grain brown rice, (e.g., Lundberg Family Farms long-grain brown jasmine rice)

¼ cup cooked short-grain brown rice

1 cup drained and rinsed black beans

½–1 teaspoon coarse kosher salt

½ teaspoon freshly cracked black pepper

¼ cup chopped fresh cilantro

⅛ cup brown rice syrup

½ cup ground sunflower seeds (this can be done in a blender or food processor)

2 tablespoons sorghum flour

Olive oil, for frying

- If you prefer, you can sauté the onion and garlic before mixing with the other ingredients, but that's up to you. Place all of the ingredients (except oil) in a large bowl and mix very well. To make these burgers hold together, you almost need to knead the mixture.

- Heat a large skillet over medium-high heat and pour in a small amount of oil. Take about ½ cup of the mixture and form it into a ball. Place the ball on the skillet and press it into a patty. Fry over medium-high heat on each side until crisp but not burned—watch that heat! It will take approximately 5 minutes on each side to cook. If you undercook the patty, it will fall apart, so make sure it is browned, then flip and cook the other side. Transfer to a platter and continue cooking the patties until you have made them all.

VEGGIE-STUFFED BELL PEPPERS

This recipe typically makes more than you can fit into four bell peppers. When I was creating the recipe, I had extra filling, so I used it as the filling for Eggplant Roll-Ups (page 88). Try both recipes; I think you will enjoy them, and what a great way to use up your leftovers!

1 tablespoon extra-virgin olive oil

½ cup finely chopped red or yellow onion

½ cup chopped zucchini

10 cremini or other mushrooms, cleaned and chopped (about ¼ pound)

4 cloves garlic, chopped finely

½ cup white wine

1 cup cooked brown or wild rice mix

¼ cup chopped walnuts, pine nuts, almonds, or pecans

1 teaspoon herbes de Provence (start with 1 teaspoon and go up to 2 teaspoons, if you wish; I like more!)

½–1 teaspoon coarse kosher salt

½ teaspoon freshly cracked black pepper, or less if desired

4 large red, green, yellow, or orange bell peppers

- Preheat the oven to 350°F.
- Heat a large skillet over medium heat. Pour in the olive oil and sauté the onion for about 3 minutes. Add the zucchini, mushrooms, and garlic, and continue to cook for 4 to 5 minutes longer. Add the wine, the cooked rice, walnuts, herbs, salt, and pepper. Mix together well. Turn off the heat and set aside.
- To prepare the peppers, cut off the stem end and wash them, inside and out. Be sure to remove the seeds in the middle, then fill the peppers with the vegetable mixture. Fill them all the way to the top, pressing down to add more so they are well filled. Place the stuffed peppers in a large baking dish, sitting them upright. Add about ¼ cup of water to the bottom of the baking dish. Bake for about 30 minutes. The peppers should be soft, so if they are not, add another 5 to 10 minutes. You don't want them to collapse, so check them after the additional 5 minutes. Serve hot.

YAM ENCHILADAS WITH POMEGRANATE SAUCE

This recipe was given to me by a very special friend, Lewis Perkin. It is printed with his permission. He is a very talented vegetarian chef and I am honored that he shared this recipe with all of us.

3 large yams

1 medium-size yellow onion, chopped

4 cloves garlic, chopped

1 tablespoon crushed coriander seeds

1 tablespoon cumin seeds

1 chopped jalapeño, for extra-spicy version

1 tablespoon cocoa powder

1 tablespoon chile powder

1 teaspoon organic brown sugar

2 tablespoons dried oregano

1 (14-ounce) can crushed tomatoes

Seeds and juice from 1 pomegranate

I tablespoon heated corn oil (optional)

4 large corn tortillas

■ Preheat the oven to 350°F. Bake the yams until soft (45 minutes to an hour). Do not turn off the oven when the yams are removed.

■ Meanwhile, sauté the onion in a large skillet over medium heat until transparent. Add the garlic, cumin, and coriander seeds, and continue to sauté for 5 minutes (adding the chopped jalapeño for the extra-spicy version) Add the cocoa, chile powder, brown sugar, and oregano, and cook for another 5 minutes. Add the tomatoes and the pomegranate seeds and juice. Simmer for at least 20 more minutes, adding water as necessary to create a medium-thick sauce.

■ Slice the yams in half, scoop out the cooked yam from its skins, and place in a warm bowl. Dip the tortillas in the hot corn oil (or wrap in foil in a warm oven) until limp. Fill each tortilla with cooked yam and roll into an enchilada shape. Cover the bottom of an 9 × 11-inch baking dish with enough of this sauce to coat the bottom of the pan. Place in the baking pan and cover with the remaining sauce. Raise the oven temperature to 375°F. Bake the enchiladas for 10 to 15 minutes.

BREAKFAST FOODS

BLUEBERRY BUCKWHEAT PANCAKES

BREAKFAST RICE WITH FRUIT

BREAKFAST RISOTTO

BREAKFAST VEGETABLE BAKE

COCONUT PANCAKES

GRANOLA

POTATO AND TOFU HASH

TOFU SCRAMBLE

BLUEBERRY BUCKWHEAT PANCAKES

SERVES 4

I love these. Serve them with the maple butter, berry sauce, Mango Madness Sauce (page 175), or your favorite jam. They are filling and good for you.

1 tablespoon Ener-G egg replacer whisked together with 4 tablespoons warm water

1½ cup hemp or soy milk

2 tablespoons grapeseed oil, plus extra for frying

2 tablespoons maple syrup

¼ cup applesauce

¾ cup buckwheat flour

½ cup brown rice flour

2 teaspoons baking powder

1 teaspoon cinnamon

1 cup blueberries

■ In a medium-size bowl, whisk the egg replacer and water well, until it bubbles and the powder is completely dissolved. Add the milk, oil, and maple syrup. Mix well. Add the applesauce and stir.

■ In a small bowl, stir together the buckwheat and brown rice flours, baking powder, and cinnamon. Add the dry mixture to the wet mixture. Stir, then incorporate the blueberries.

■ Heat a skillet over medium-high heat. Pour in a small amount of oil. When the skillet is hot, pour in a ladleful of batter. Cook until done, flipping halfway through the cooking process. If your batter is too thick, add a small amount of milk or water to thin it out.

BREAKFAST RICE WITH FRUIT

What a great way to use up leftovers and eat healthy. You could use other fruits, but this was what I had in my refrigerator the day I developed this recipe. Try peaches, or nectarines, or blueberries. The sky's the limit!

2 cups soy, almond, rice, or coconut milk

2 cups leftover cooked rice (brown preferred)

1 large apple, chopped (about 1½ cups)

¼ cup agave nectar

½ teaspoon cinnamon

½ cup currants or raisins

¼ cup walnuts or your choice of nuts

Pinch of salt

■ Heat the milk in a 4-quart saucepan. Add all the ingredients and heat through. Season with salt and serve.

BREAKFAST RISOTTO

SERVES 4

We all know breakfast is the most important meal of the day, but so many people skip it or eat junk. I came up with this recipe so you would have another healthy option.

1 cup uncooked Arborio rice

1 (14-ounce) can light coconut milk

2 cups water

1 (8-ounce) can pineapple chunks, drained

½ cup currants

¼ cup chopped walnuts

1 teaspoon ground cinnamon

¼ teaspoon ground cardamom

½ pitted mango or banana, peeled and chopped (optional) (See Note)

■ Pour 1 cup of water into a large skillet and place over medium heat. When it comes to a boil, add the rice. When the water is absorbed, add the other cup of water, and when that is absorbed, add 1 cup of the coconut milk. Continue cooking over medium heat until the liquid is absorbed, then add the rest of the coconut milk. When the rice is cooked and all of the liquid has been absorbed, add the pineapple, currants, nuts, spices, and, if desired, the optional fruit. Heat through, adjust seasonings, and serve.

> Note: Trader Joe's sells mangoes in the freezer section that are precut into bite-size pieces; they work well for dishes like this.

BREAKFAST VEGETABLE BAKE

SERVES 4

If you choose to use the muffin tin instead of a baking dish for this, that's fine, but be sure to add some water to any compartment that you do not fill with batter. These are easy to make and you can use several different veggies in this recipe, such as kale, cabbage, and so on.

½ cup finely chopped onion

1½ tablespoons olive oil

¾ cup cleaned, stemmed, and halved mushrooms

4 cups washed and chopped spinach

2 cloves garlic, chopped finely

1 pound extra-firm silken tofu

2 tablespoons apple juice or water

1 tablespoon chopped fresh basil

½ teaspoon sea salt

¼ teaspoon nutmeg

Freshly ground pepper

- Preheat the oven to 350°F. Lightly spray a small baking dish with vegetable oil nonstick spray, or prepare a muffin tin with the spray.
- In a large skillet, sauté the onion in the olive oil over medium-high heat until soft, 4 to 5 minutes. Add the mushrooms, spinach, and garlic, and continue to sauté for another 4 to 5 minutes.
- Meanwhile, place the tofu a blender, along with the apple juice. Puree until smooth and creamy.
- Add the tofu mixture to the skillet and continue to cook, adding the basil, sea salt, a pinch of the nutmeg, and pepper to taste.
- Pour this mixture into your prepared pan and sprinkle the rest of the nutmeg on top. Bake until lightly browned on top, 35 to 40 minutes. Serve hot.

COCONUT PANCAKES

SERVES 4 TO 6 (MAKES ABOUT 12 PANCAKES)

I sent this recipe to a family of four: Jen, Brad, Sklyer, and Zane. They agreed to be my tasters for this recipe and I got a thumbs-up: Brad left me a message and said they enjoyed them and looked forward to the new cookbook. That's a good review in my book, so you better try them, some morning, with your family. These pancakes are light in texture as well as flavor. Serve with the Mango Madness Sauce (page 175) or Berry Sauce (page 171).

1½ teaspoons Ener-G egg replacer whisked together with 2 tablespoons warm water

2 tablespoons agave nectar

1 (14-ounce) can light coconut milk

2 tablespoons unsweetened coconut

¼ cup applesauce

1½ cup sorghum flour

2 teaspoons baking powder

½ cup tapioca flour

½ teaspoon salt

2 tablespoons coconut, grapeseed, or canola oil, plus more for frying

- In a large bowl, whisk the egg replacer and water well, until it bubbles and the powder is completely dissolved. Add the other wet ingredients and beat together.
- In a separate medium-size bowl, stir all the dry ingredients together well. Add the dry ingredients to the wet ingredients and whip with a whisk until well blended. Let sit for 2 to 3 minutes while the pan heats up.
- Heat a skillet over medium-high heat. Pour in a small amount of canola oil, or spray with vegetable oil nonstick spray. Pour a ladleful of batter into the skillet.
- Cook until bubbles form and the pancake is light brown.
- Flip and cook on the other side for 2 to 3 minutes, or done. Repeat with the remaining batter.

GRANOLA

This is not just for breakfast, and I am not kidding. I use this granola in Cranberry Granola Bars (page 123). I had about ten of my taste testers try it as is, and each and every one of them loved it, and I mean *loved* it! This stuff is so good, you will want not only to eat it for breakfast but to share it as a snack, carry it with you when you travel, or serve to guests. It is addictive, so watch out!

1 cup chopped walnuts (I have also used pecans and almonds in place of the walnuts)

1 cup chopped raw cashews

½ cup pumpkin seeds

¼ cup sesame seeds

½ cup sunflower seeds

2 cups puffed rice

½ cup pitted and chopped dates (Medjool dates are the best for this)

½ tablespoon ground flax meal

1 tablespoon sorghum flour

1 teaspoon ground cinnamon

¼ teaspoon ground cardamom

¼ cup canola oil

½ cup agave nectar

- Preheat the oven to 325°F. Lightly spray a jelly-roll pan with vegetable oil nonstick spray.
- In a large bowl, combine the nuts, seeds, puffed rice, dates, flax meal, flour, and spices. Pour in the oil and agave nectar and stir to really blend everything together and distribute the nuts, seeds, and fruit evenly.
- Pour the granola into the prepared baking pan and spread it out so it covers the entire pan. Bake, uncovered, for 30 to 40 minutes, or until the mixture is a light golden brown. You must stir this during the baking process, to ensure that the granola bakes evenly.
- It will not be crunchy when you first remove it from the oven, but be careful—do not overcook. When it cools, it will become crunchy.
- As soon as it starts to cool, transfer the granola from the pan into an airtight container, and let it finish cooling there, as it is a bit sticky and may stick to the pan if it remains there. Store in the airtight container.

POTATO AND TOFU HASH

This is great for breakfast and, because it stores well, is good reheated as a leftover. I recommend that you use other vegetables, depending on the time of year. For example, I made this batch in the winter but, in the spring, you could use fresh baby carrots, new potatoes, and small zucchini, too. I like to adjust recipes to the seasons. Give it a try.

1–2 tablespoons grapeseed or canola oil

1 large red onion, chopped (about 1 cup)

1 medium-size red bell pepper, seeded and chopped

4 medium-size red potatoes, scrubbed, peeled if desired, grated, and patted dry

½ cup fresh or frozen peas (never canned!)

½ pound extra-firm tofu (preferably silken, but any will do), crumbled

2 tablespoons drained and finely chopped sun-dried tomatoes

½ teaspoon coarse salt

¼ teaspoon freshly ground pepper

1 teaspoon rosemary (optional)

Salsa (optional)

■ Heat a large skillet over medium-high heat and pour in the oil. Add the onions and red bell pepper, and sauté until the onion becomes soft, 4 to 5 minutes. Add the potatoes and continue to cook over medium-high heat for 10 to 15 minutes, or until the potatoes begin to brown. Add the peas and tofu, and cook for an additional 5 minutes. Add the tomatoes and heat through. Season with lots of freshly ground pepper and the salt, and, if desired, the rosemary. Serve with salsa, if desired.

TOFU SCRAMBLE

SERVES 4

Here's another option for breakfast. I teach cooking classes and many times I hear folks complain that it's hard to find something healthy for breakfast. Well, try this. This tastes just as good heated up as it does when you first make it.

2 tablespoons olive oil

1 large onion (about 1 cup), chopped

½ cup sliced carrots

½ cup seeded and chopped red bell pepper

1 cup chopped zucchini

1 cup cleaned and chopped mushrooms (optional)

2 cloves garlic, chopped

1 cup seeded and diced organic tomatoes

1 pound tofu, drained and cut into cubes (I prefer extra-firm silken)

2 teaspoons wheat-free tamari sauce

1 teaspoon curry powder

Freshly ground pepper

■ Place the oil in a large skillet and heat over medium-high heat. Add the onion and sauté until soft, 3 to 4 minutes. Add the carrots, and continue to cook for 2 to 3 minutes. Add the red bell pepper, zucchini, and mushrooms, and sauté for 2 minutes. Add the garlic and cook for 1 minute. Add the tomatoes, tofu, tamari sauce, and curry powder, and stir to mix well. Cook until heated through and the vegetables are fork tender. The flavors should be blended well. Serve immediately.

BREADS, MUFFINS, SCONES, AND CRUSTS

BAKING POWDER BISCUITS

CARROT BREAD

CORNBREAD

CRANBERRY GRANOLA BARS

CURRANT SCONES

DOSAS

FRESH UNCOOKED PIECRUST

GINGERBREAD

OAT SCONES

PIECRUST

PIZZA CRUST

PUMPKIN SCONES

BAKING POWDER BISCUITS

These are not easy to make without gluten. I have done my best, and I think you will enjoy them, but they won't last long. They are best eaten fresh, as they dry out within a day or two.

¾ cup brown rice flour

1 tablespoon organic sugar

1 tablespoon baking powder

¼ teaspoon salt

¼ cup coconut shortening or palm oil

¼ cup hemp or soy milk

■ Preheat the oven to 375°F.

■ Place the brown rice flour, sugar, baking powder, and salt in a large mixing bowl. Using a pastry cutter or fork, cut in the shortening until mixed. Add the milk and stir to form a ball. Scatter some brown rice flour on a work surface and knead the dough a few times, then press or roll out the dough until it is about ½ inch thick. Using a 2-inch glass or biscuit cutter, gently cut out the biscuits and place on a cooking sheet. Bake for 10 to 12 minutes, or until lightly browned on the bottom. Cool on a wire rack. Serve with jam or maple butter.

CARROT BREAD

MAKES 1 LOAF

I took this around town to about ten different people to taste. Everyone wanted the recipe immediately. They just raved about it, so I hope you enjoy it as much as they did!

½ cup canola oil

¾ cup agave nectar

1 tablespoon Ener-G egg replacer whisked together with ¼ cup warm water

¼ cup unsweetened applesauce

1 cup brown rice flour

½ cup quinoa flour

2 teaspoons baking powder

1 teaspoon baking soda

½ teaspoon sea salt

1 teaspoon ground cinnamon

1 teaspoon xanthan gum

¼ cup chopped walnuts

½ cup pitted and chopped dates

1 cup grated carrots

¼ cup crushed pineapple, drained

- Preheat the oven to 350°F. Lightly grease a 9 × 5 × 3-inch loaf pan with vegetable oil.
- In a large mixing bowl, beat the oil and agave nectar together until mixture is smooth and well blended. In a small bowl, whisk the egg replacer with the warm water, until bubbles form and the powder has completely dissolved. Add this mixture to the agave mixture and stir. Stir in the applesauce.
- In another bowl combine the brown rice and quinoa flours, baking powder, baking soda, salt, cinnamon, and xanthan gum, and stir. Add the flour mixture to the agave mixture and stir together really well. Add the walnuts, dates, carrots, and pineapple. Stir well, then spoon the batter into the prepared loaf pan. The batter will be thick.
- Bake for 50 minutes, or until a toothpick or sharp knife inserted in the middle comes out clean. Cool on a wire rack, then remove from pan. Enjoy.

CORNBREAD

This cornbread can be stored in an airtight container for several days. I like it served with the black beans or alongside J&J's Favorite Yam and Black Bean Burritos (page 91; leave out the tortilla and just serve with the cornbread).

1½ teaspoons Ener-G egg replacer whisked together with 2 tablespoons warm water

¼ cup agave nectar

¼ cup grapeseed oil

1 cup hemp or soy milk

½ cup brown rice flour

½ cup sorghum flour

4 teaspoons baking powder

½ teaspoon sea salt

1 cup cornmeal

- Preheat the oven to 425°F. Spray an 8- or 9-inch square pan with vegetable oil nonstick spray.
- In a small bowl, whisk the egg replacer with the warm water, until bubbles form and the powder has completely dissolved.
- In a large mixing bowl, combine the agave nectar and oil, and beat until smooth and thick, 1 to 2 minutes. Add the egg replacer mixture and hemp milk, and continue to mix until well blended.
- In a separate bowl, combine the brown rice and sorghum flours, baking powder, salt, and cornmeal, and stir well together. Add the flour mixture to the liquid mixture and stir just until it becomes incorporated. Do not overbeat. Pour into the prepared baking pan and bake until lightly browned on top, 18 to 20 minutes. Cool on a wire rack and serve. This is wonderful served as an accompaniment to black beans, with a side of guacamole.

CRANBERRY GRANOLA BARS

MAKES ABOUT 24

These are yummy, yummy in the tummy! I can't say enough about these. I once had a recipe for cranberry granola bars that were made with sugar, butter, white flour, and eggs. The following bars are so good and their ingredients are so much better than the ones made with those other ingredients! I have made these with organic brown sugar and agave. I prefer agave, but you be the judge!

1½ teaspoons Ener-G egg replacer whisked together with 2 tablespoons warm water

¼ cup canola oil

¾ cup organic brown sugar or agave nectar

¼ cup applesauce

½ cup sorghum flour

½ cup brown rice flour

2 teaspoons baking powder

½ teaspoon salt

2 cups homemade granola (page 115)

1 cup dried cranberries, or currants or raisins

- Preheat the oven to 350°F. Lightly spray a 9-inch square baking dish with vegetable oil non-stick spray.
- In a small bowl, whisk the egg replacer with the warm water, until bubbles form and the powder has completely dissolved.
- In a large mixing bowl, combine the oil and brown sugar. Beat well, then add the applesauce and egg replacer mixture. Continue to beat until well blended. Add the sorghum and brown rice flours, baking powder, and salt, and mix together well. Add the granola and cranberries, and stir to incorporate them into the batter.
- Pour the batter (this is thick, so don't expect it to really "pour") into the prepared pan and bake for 30 to 35 minutes, or until done. Check for doneness 25 to 30 minutes into the baking process. These are sticky, so they won't be completely "clean" when you check on them. Cool on a wire rack.

CURRANT SCONES

I really like scones and there are so many things you can do with them. Depending on the time of year, you can add berries or other ingredients. I encourage you to be creative and make these first as written, and then to try something new with them next time—add a new spice, or a new fruit. Dried cranberries, blueberries, or nuts can be substituted for the currants or raisins.

2 tablespoons agave nectar

4 tablespoons vegan margarine

1½ teaspoons Ener-G egg replacer whisked together with 2 tablespoons warm water

¼ cup applesauce

½ cup soy, almond, rice, or hemp milk

1½ cups sorghum flour

½ cup tapioca flour

¼ cup brown rice flour

2 tablespoons arrowroot powder

2 teaspoons baking powder

½ teaspoon baking soda

1 teaspoon xanthan gum

½ teaspoon salt

1 teaspoon ground cardamom

½ cup currants or raisins

- Preheat the oven to 375°F. Line a cookie sheet with baking parchment or grease the pan.
- In a large bowl, blend together the margarine and agave nectar until light and creamy.
- In a small bowl, whisk the egg replacer with the warm water, until bubbles form and the powder has completely dissolved.
- Add this mixture to the agave mixture along with the applesauce and stir well. Add the milk and continue stirring. The mixture will appear curdled.
- Sift together all of the dry ingredients, with the exception of the currants or raisins. Add dry ingredients to the wet ingredients. Beat until just blended. Do not overbeat. Stir in the currants or raisins to incorporate.
- Press out the mixture on a cutting board, forming a round shape about ½ inch thick. Cut into eight triangles and place on the prepared cookie sheet. Bake until lightly browned, 12 to 15 minutes. Cool on a wire rack.

DOSAS

These are like mini pancakes, but they don't cook like pancakes. Don't expect them to produce little bubbles when it's time to flip them over. That won't happen. You need to keep your eyes ready for dryness: that's the time to flip them over, when the edges begin to dry out. I use grapeseed oil for frying because it can withstand high heat.

2 cups brown rice flour
½ cup quinoa flour
3 cups water
½ teaspoon salt
Grapeseed oil, for frying

- Place the brown rice and quinoa flours, water, and salt in a large bowl and beat until very well blended. The ingredients have a tendency to separate, so whisk them together well before you prepare to cook them.

- Heat a large skillet over high heat and pour in a little grapeseed oil. When it is hot, add a small ladleful of batter to the skillet. The diameter of the pancake should be no larger than 7 to 8 inches across. Cook until the dosa begins to become dry around the edges. Unlike cooking a pancake, which is still very wet on top when you turn it, you want to be sure the dosa is cooked through before you flip it, so let it cook for a few minutes and, when the edges look dry, then flip it and cook the other side. If the dosa begins to burn, reduce the heat slightly. Place each dosa on a cooling rack or between waxed paper until you have cooked the entire batch. Fill with your favorite filling. I like to use Spinach Dal (page 76).

FRESH UNCOOKED PIECRUST

This crust can be used with several recipes in this book: Raspberry Tofu Pudding (page 153) or Chocolate Pudding (142) are good fillings. Tropical Pudding or Pie Filling (page 155) is also great made with this crust.

4 cups walnuts or raw
  macadamia nuts
1½ cups pitted Medjool dates
¼ teaspoon ground cinnamon
⅛ teaspoon ground ginger
Pinch of freshly grated nutmeg
Pinch of ground cardamom
¼ teaspoon salt

■ Place all of the nuts into a food processor or, if necessary, a blender and process until fine. (If you are using a blender, be sure to chop all the nuts and dates before putting them into the machine. Blenders are not the best tool for this job, because you want the mixture to be fine, and unless you do very small batches, it will be challenging to achieve this using a blender.) Add the dates and continue to process until the mixture is well blended, and no large particles remain. Add the spices and salt, and blend to mix together. Lightly grease a pie dish with vegetable oil nonstick spray and press the mixture into the dish, using your hands, pressing the dough evenly onto the bottom of the dish and up the sides.

Note: If you want to vary your crust, try using 2 cups walnuts and 2 cups pecans or macadamia nuts. I also use pecans in this crust with great results.

GINGERBREAD

This is the best thing next to Grandma's. Kids love it and adults do, too. I made some today and put a tiny bit of maple butter on it and it was wonderful. This stores well and also freezes well.

¼ cup vegan margarine

½ cup agave nectar

¼ cup molasses

½ teaspoon vanilla extract

1½ teaspoons Ener-G egg replacer whisked together with 2 tablespoons warm water

2 teaspoons orange rind

⅛ cup soy or hemp milk

1 cup applesauce

1 teaspoon crystallized ginger

¾ cup sorghum flour

¾ cup brown rice flour

2 teaspoons baking powder

2 teaspoons ground ginger

½ teaspoon salt

1 teaspoon ground cinnamon

2 teaspoon xanthan gum

- Preheat the oven to 350°F. Lightly spray a 9-inch square baking dish with vegetable oil non-stick spray.
- Place the margarine and agave nectar in a large mixing bowl and beat to combine well. Add the molasses and vanilla, and continue beating.
- In a small bowl, whisk the egg replacer with the warm water, until bubbles form and the powder has completely dissolved. Add to the margarine mixture the egg replacer mixture, orange rind, milk, applesauce, and crystallized ginger, and stir.
- In a separate bowl, sift together the sorghum flour, brown rice flour, baking powder, ground ginger, salt, cinnamon, and xanthan gum. Add the dry ingredients to the wet ingredients and stir together until they are well incorporated.
- Pour the ingredients into the prepared baking dish. Bake until lightly browned and a toothpick inserted in the middle comes out clean, about 25 minutes. Cool on a wire rack.

OAT SCONES

MAKES 8

Oats have long been a concern for people suffering with celiac disease because the oats were processed in the same manufacturing plants as were other glutinous products. Today gluten-free oats are available (check out www.glutenfreeoats.com or www. giftsofnature.net), so those who want to eat oats can do so without worrying. These scones are wonderful served with maple butter.

⅓ cup canola oil

2 tablespoons agave nectar

2 tablespoons warm water

1 tablespoon orange juice

½ cup sorghum flour (or more as needed)

1 teaspoon baking soda

¼ teaspoon salt

⅓ cup pitted dates

⅓ cup rolled oats

- Preheat the oven to 325°F.
- In a large mixing bowl, combine the oil and agave nectar, and beat well. Add the water and orange juice, and stir well. Scatter a tablespoon or two of oats across an ungreased cookie sheet.
- In a small bowl, stir together the sorghum flour, baking soda, and salt. Stir into the oil mixture. Add the dates and stir. Beat with a wooden spoon until well mixed.
- Add additional sorghum flour until you can form a ball. The dough should not be really sticky.
- Place about ¼ cup of the oats on a work surface. Roll or press the ball of dough into the oats until it becomes a 5–inch-diameter circle about ½ inch thick. Place on the prepared pan. Bake at for 20 to 25 minutes, or until lightly browned. Cool on the cookie sheet and serve.

PIECRUST

This crust takes some effort, but it is worth it. I used it for Apple-Raspberry Pie (page 135), and the bottom didn't get soggy; the pie tasted like a regular pie. Now, that's amazing!

1½ cups brown rice flour

½ cup arrowroot

½ teaspoon salt

1 teaspoon xanthan gum

¼ cup potato starch

½ cup vegan shortening

1 tablespoon white vinegar

½ cup + 2 tablespoons cold water

■ Place all of the dry ingredients in a large mixing bowl and stir well. Cut in the shortening until it is well blended, then add the vinegar and water a little at a time. Keep adding the water and mixing well until you have a dough that you can push together into a ball. This takes time, but keep at it—you really have to work at this dough, but you will be very glad you did—several times before you roll it out, so it will really stick together. Break into two equal balls.

■ Spread a large piece of waxed paper on your surface area. Place one of the balls on the paper and press flat. Cover with another large piece of waxed paper and use a rolling pin to roll out into the size you need to fit into a 9-inch pie dish. Before you put the dough in the pie dish, spray the dish lightly with vegetable oil nonstick spray so the crust won't stick. Then, carefully pull off the top piece of waxed paper and gently flip the rolled-out dough over into the pie dish. Once you have it positioned correctly, carefully (again) lift the remaining waxed paper off the dough. Spoon your filling in the piecrust and then roll out the second crust and place it in the above manner on top of the pie filling. Carefully remove the waxed paper, and pinch the dough all the way around to join the top and bottom crust, so the filling will not spill out during the baking process. Bake according to the cooking instructions provided for your pie filling. Cool on a wire rack.

Breads, Muffins, Scones, and Crusts 129

ZA CRUST

This crust is what I have used for both of the pizza recipes in this book (pages 94 and 177). It isn't as easy to work as with traditional pizza dough but stick with it; you will be happy you did.

1 cup Bob's Red Mill All-Purpose GF Baking Flour

¼ cup potato flour

2 teaspoons baking powder

½ teaspoon sea salt

½ teaspoon xanthan gum

1½ teaspoons Ener-G egg replacer whisked together with 2 tablespoons warm water

1 tablespoon agave nectar

½ cup hemp or soy milk

⅛ cup grapeseed or canola oil

- Preheat the oven to 400°F. Grease a pizza or jelly-roll pan lightly with a vegetable oil nonstick spray.
- In a large bowl, combine the GF baking and potato flours, baking powder, salt, and xanthan gum. Mix well.
- In a small bowl, whisk the egg replacer with the warm water, until bubbles form and the powder has completely dissolved. Add the agave nectar to this mixture, as well as the hemp milk and grapeseed oil. Whisk together and add to the dry ingredients. Stir with a wooden spoon to mix well.
- Flatten out the pizza dough on the prepared pan until it is evenly spread across the entire surface. Top with your favorite veggies and bake until done, about 15 minutes. Check the pizza after about 12 minutes and continue to monitor it until it is heated through and the crust is crisp. Cool on a wire rack.

PUMPKIN SCONES

MAKES 8

I love anything made with pumpkin, any time of year. You will enjoy these, and I know your children will, too. These store well in a airtight container for several days. They also freeze well. These are great served with maple butter.

¾ cup brown rice flour

½ cup sorghum flour

1 teaspoon xanthan gum

2 teaspoons baking powder

1 teaspoon baking soda

¼ cup arrowroot powder

¼ cup potato starch

½ teaspoon ground cinnamon

¼ teaspoon grated nutmeg

½ teaspoon sea salt

6 tablespoons vegan margarine

1½ teaspoons Ener-G egg replacer whisked together with 2 tablespoons warm water

2 tablespoons agave nectar

⅓ cup hemp or soy milk

½ teaspoon vanilla extract

¾ cup pureed pumpkin

- Preheat the oven to 425°F.
- In a large bowl, combine the brown rice and sorghum flours, xanthan gum, baking powder, baking soda, arrowroot powder, potato starch, cinnamon, nutmeg, and salt. Stir to mix well. Add the margarine, cutting it into the dry ingredients until it is fully incorporated. The mixture should resemble small peas.
- In a small bowl, whisk the egg replacer with the warm water, until bubbles form and the powder has completely dissolved. Add the agave nectar, hemp milk, and vanilla, and whisk together well. Add the pumpkin and stir well. Add this mixture to the dry ingredients and mix it all together, but do not overbeat.
- Lightly flour a work surface. Place the dough on the surface, then pat or roll it out until about it is ½ to ¾ inch thick. Cut into wedges and place carefully on a cookie sheet. Bake for 15 to 20 minutes, or until browned. Keep an eye on them as they bake so they don't become too dark.
- Cool on a wire rack. Store in an airtight container or freeze.

DESSERTS

APPLE PIE BARS

APPLE-RASPBERRY PIE FILLING

AWESOME NO-BAKE CHOCOLATE COOKIES

BERRY AND CHERRY CRISP

BROWNIES

BUTTERNUT SQUASH DESSERT

CARROT CAKE

CHOCOLATE CHIP COOKIES

CHOCOLATE PUDDING

COCONUT RICE PUDDING

CRISPY RICE TREATS, HEALTHY STYLE

DELICIOUS BAKED APPLES

FROZEN BANANAS

GINGER RICE PUDDING

PEACH AND BLUEBERRY COBBLER

PEANUT BUTTER CANDY

PEANUT BUTTER COOKIES

PEAR TORTE

QUINOA COFFEE CAKE

RASPBERRY TOFU PUDDING

SUPER-DUPER FUDGE

TROPICAL PUDDING OR PIE FILLING

APPLE PIE BARS

These are a real treat. They do take some time to make, but they are worth the effort, I assure you. I have made these bars with both agave cactus nectar and brown rice syrup. My taste testers liked it best with the agave but, either way, they are delicious.

Crust

2½ cups sorghum flour

1 teaspoon salt

1 teaspoon xanthan gum

6 tablespoons vegan margarine (Earth Balance is a great brand)

1½ teaspoons Ener-G egg replacer whisked together with 2 tablespoons warm water

Rice or soy milk

Filling

1 cup corn flakes or millet flakes, crushed

4–6 large apples, peeled, cored, and sliced thinly

1 tablespoon sorghum flour

1 cup agave nectar or brown rice syrup

1½ teaspoons ground cinnamon

½ teaspoon grated nutmeg

- Preheat the oven to 350°F. Lightly spray a jelly-roll pan or large cookie sheet with vegetable oil nonstick spray.
- Place the flour, salt, and xanthan gum in a large mixing bowl. Cut in the margarine until crumbly. Set aside.
- In a small bowl, whisk the egg replacer with the warm water, until bubbles form and the powder has completely dissolved. Add enough milk to equal ⅔ cup liquid. Pour the wet mixture over the dry mixture and mix together well. You should be able to form the dough into a ball. Knead four or five times to really bind it together. Break the ball in half.
- Place a piece of waxed paper (about 13 × 10 inches) on a cutting board or counter. Place half the dough on the waxed paper and cover it with another piece of waxed paper cut to the same size. Using a rolling pin, roll out the ball until it is 13 × 10. Carefully remove the top layer of paper from the dough. Gently turn the dough onto a prepared pan and remove the remaining layer of waxed paper. Spread the crushed cereal over the top of the dough.
- Layer the apples over the cereal, to the edges of the dough. In a small bowl, mix the agave nectar, sorghum flour, cinnamon, and nutmeg. Pour this mixture over the apples.
- Roll out the other ball of dough exactly as you did the first one, and gently lay this over the top of the apples. Make sure you cover as much as you can of the bottom layer.
- Sprinkle with extra cinnamon, if desired, and bake for about 45 minutes, or until bubbly. (Baste the top with juices from the apples and agave nectar during the baking process, two or three times.) Cut into bars and serve.

APPLE-RASPBERRY PIE FILLING

This is a great pie. If you use my recipe for piecrust (page 129), you will be amazed at how good this tastes. I have given this recipe to people who are not vegans or do not eat gluten free, and they loved it.

1 double-crust piecrust (page 129, or your preferred recipe)

5 cups peeled or unpeeled, cored, thinly sliced apples

3 cups raspberries

1 cup agave nectar

1 teaspoon ground cinnamon

Pinch of sea salt

6 tablespoons sorghum flour

- Preheat the oven to 350°F. Place the bottom crust of the piecrust dough in a pie pan.
- Place the apples in a large mixing bowl and add the rest of the ingredients. Toss to coat well.
- Pour this mixture into the piecrust and top with the second crust as described on page 129. Bake until lightly browned, about 55 minutes. Cool on a wire rack.

AWESOME NO-BAKE CHOCOLATE COOKIES

MAKES 1 DOZEN

These uncooked cookies are very good but rich. Savor them, don't gobble them. They are divinely decadent.

½ cup coconut

2 cups vegan chocolate chips (Enjoy Life Foods makes wonderful vegan chips!)

½ cup pitted, finely chopped Medjool dates

¼ cup finely chopped pecans or walnuts

¼ cup almond, cashew, or macadamia/cashew butter

2 tablespoons brown rice syrup or agave nectar

1 teaspoon vanilla extract

⅛ teaspoon ground cinnamon

- Prepare a large platter by lining it with baking parchment.
- Toast the coconut: Heat a small skillet on the burner over medium-high heat. When the skillet is hot, add the coconut and, with a wooden spoon or spatula, stir it around in the pan until it starts to brown. Don't let it burn, just toast it lightly. Remove from the heat and set aside.
- Meanwhile, melt the chocolate in a double boiler and, when it has melted, place it in a large bowl to cool slightly. Add the rest of the ingredients including the coconut, and mix until thoroughly blended.
- Drop by spoonfuls on the prepared platter, and refrigerate until completely cooled.

BERRY AND CHERRY CRISP

SERVES 8

I have always been a crisp lover. I prefer fruit over chocolate, any day. This is a great dessert to take along to a picnic or party, or to have for dessert during the heat of the summer. You can also use apples, peaches, blackberries, strawberries . . . whatever you prefer. Just remember to swap out equal amounts for the fruits here.

Topping

½ cup brown rice flour or sorghum flour

½ cup certified gluten-free oats

½ cup chopped walnuts

½ cup organic brown sugar

1 teaspoon ground cinnamon

¼ cup vegan margarine

Filling

3 cups raspberries

3½ pounds cherries, stemmed and pitted

3 tablespoons arrowroot powder

1 cup agave nectar or organic brown sugar

1 teaspoon vanilla extract

2 tablespoons lemon juice

- Preheat the oven to 375°F. Have ready a 9 × 13-inch rectangular baking dish.
- Prepare the topping: Place the brown rice flour, oats, walnuts, brown sugar, and cinnamon in a medium-size bowl and stir together. Cut in the margarine and keep working on this until the mixture is well incorporated. You can use a fork, your fingers, or a pastry cutter to blend the dough. Set aside.
- Prepare the filling: Heat the raspberries, cherries, arrowroot, and agave nectar in a large saucepan. Stir often so the mixture does not stick to the bottom of the pan. When it comes to a boil, add the vanilla and lemon juice, then lower the heat and cook for 1 to 2 minutes, or until the mixture thickens. If your fruit is really juicy, the mixture may not thicken, and you will need to add another tablespoon of arrowroot. Pour the mixture into the baking dish and spread the topping evenly over the fruit mixture. Bake until the fruit is bubbling and the topping is browned, 40 to 45 minutes. (Oven temperatures vary, so check on this at 35 minutes. You don't want your topping to burn.)
- Serve either hot or cold.

BROWNIES

MAKES 24

My friends were hesitant to believe that I could come up with a gluten-free, vegan brownie, but guess who got the last laugh? These are great and you will be surprised at how quickly they will disappear.

¼ cup oil

1½ cups organic sugar

1 cup applesauce

1 banana, peeled and mashed

1½ teaspoons Ener-G egg replacer whisked together with 2 tablespoons warm water

1 cup cocoa powder

½ cup brown rice flour

½ cup quinoa flour

2 teaspoons baking powder

1 teaspoon xanthan gum

¼ teaspoon salt

½ cup vegan chocolate chips

¼ cup chopped walnuts

- Preheat the oven to 350°F. Spray an 8-inch square pan with vegetable oil nonstick spray.

- In a large mixing bowl, beat together the oil and organic sugar. Since there is such a small amount of oil, this will not become light and fluffy, but mix it together for a minute or two, then add the applesauce, mashed banana, and egg replacer, and beat for 1 to 2 minutes. (Be sure you whisk the egg replacer very well with the warm water until it is bubbly and the powder has dissolved.) Add the cocoa and stir to blend.

- In a separate bowl, sift together the brown rice and quinoa flours, baking powder, xanthan gum, and salt. Add to the wet ingredients and mix together until well blended. Add the chocolate chips and walnuts, and stir by hand to incorporate. Do not overbeat.

- Spoon the batter into the prepared pan. Spread it around evenly, then bake for 35 to 40 minutes. Because these brownies are very much like real brownies, you don't want them to get dried out in the baking process, so when you test them, don't expect the toothpick or knife to come out completely clean. It won't, due to the melted chocolate chips. Cool on a wire rack, then cut into bars.

BUTTERNUT SQUASH DESSERT

SERVES 6

I developed this recipe for a gluten-free cooking class that I was teaching. The participants loved it and all asked for the recipe. It is refreshing, and because I love raspberries, that's what I included here, but you could use blueberries, blackberries, or strawberries, and it would be just as good.

1 small butternut squash

1 tablespoon grapeseed or olive oil

6 ounces extra-firm silken tofu

¼ cup maple syrup or agave nectar

⅓ cup orange juice, freshly squeezed if possible

½ cup hemp or coconut milk

2 tablespoons grated orange zest

2 cups fresh raspberries

⅛ teaspoon grated nutmeg

- Preheat the oven to 400°F. Cut the ends off of the butternut squash, then cut in half lengthwise. Scoop out the seeds, and brush the cut sides of the squash with the oil. Place on a large cookie sheet, cut side down, and roast until tender, about 45 minutes. As soon as the squash is tender (poke it with a fork), remove from the oven and cool.

- Scoop out enough of the squash to equal 1 cup. Place it a food processor or blender. Add the tofu, maple syrup, orange juice, hemp milk, and orange zest. Blend until completely smooth.

- Place the fresh berries in a serving dish and top with the squash mixture. Sprinkle the nutmeg on top and chill for at least 30 minutes. Serve cold.

CARROT CAKE

This cake is great to take to a party or pot luck. Frost with the Cashew Crème Frosting (page 171) if you want. I like it without a frosting, but if you are making it for a birthday party, you might want to frost it.

½ cup canola oil

1 cup organic brown sugar or agave nectar

1½ teaspoons Ener-G egg replacer whisked together with 2 tablespoons warm water

½ cup applesauce

1½ teaspoons vanilla extract

3–4 large carrots, grated (about 1½ cups)

¾ cup crushed pineapple, drained

1 cup brown rice flour

½ cup quinoa flour

2 teaspoons baking powder

1 teaspoon baking soda

1½ teaspoons ground cinnamon

½ teaspoon grated nutmeg

½ teaspoon salt

1 teaspoon xanthan gum

¾ cup chopped walnuts

⅓ cup unsweetened coconut (optional)

Cashew Crème Frosting (optional)

- Preheat the oven to 350°F. Lightly spray a 9 × 11-inch rectangular baking dish with vegetable oil nonstick spray.
- In a large mixing bowl, combine the oil and organic brown sugar. Beat on high for a few minutes, until the mixture becomes thick and creamy. Add the egg replacer mixture, applesauce, and vanilla, and stir to blend well. Add the carrots and pineapple, and stir.
- In a smaller bowl, sift together the brown rice and quinoa flours, baking powder, baking soda, cinnamon, nutmeg, salt, and xanthan gum. Add the dry mixture to the wet mixture and beat until well incorporated. Add the walnuts and coconut, and stir well.
- Pour the batter into the prepared baking dish and bake until done, 30 to 35 minutes. Using a toothpick or a clean, sharp knife, test the cake at the 20-minute mark, as oven temperatures vary and you don't want the cake to become too dry. The tester should come out clean with no sign of raw batter. This is a very moist cake, so be careful not to overbake.
- Cool on a wire rack and serve with Cashew Crème Frosting, if desired.

CHOCOLATE CHIP COOKIES

MAKES ABOUT 3 DOZEN

These are great cookies and if you keep them in an airtight container they will last several days. You can also put them in a zipper-top plastic bag and freeze them for later. It might be a good idea to do that, because if you have them around, they may get eaten sooner, rather than later.

1 cup vegan margarine

1 cup agave nectar

1 teaspoon vanilla extract

1 tablespoon Ener-G egg replacer whisked together with 4 tablespoons warm water

1½ cups sorghum flour

½ cup tapioca flour

½ cup garbanzo bean flour

1 teaspoon xanthan gum

2 teaspoons baking powder

1 teaspoon baking soda

½ teaspoon ground cinnamon

½ teaspoon sea salt

1 cup vegan chocolate chips

¼ cup sesame seeds or chopped nuts

- Preheat the oven to 350°F. Line a cookie sheet with baking parchment or spray lightly with vegetable oil nonstick spray. In a large mixing bowl, combine the margarine with the agave nectar and beat well, so the mixture is fully creamed together. Add the vanilla and egg replacer mixture, and stir to mix.

- In another bowl, sift together the sorghum, tapioca, and garbanzo bean flours, xanthan gum, baking powder, baking soda, cinnamon, and salt. Add the dry mixture to the wet mixture and mix well. Add the chocolate chips and sesame seeds, and stir together well.

- Drop by spoonfuls onto the prepared cookie sheet. Bake for 15 to 18 minutes. Cool on a wire rack.

> **Note: If you find that these cookies are too crumbly, add 1 additional teaspoon of xanthan gum. I like them as they are, buy you decide!**

CHOCOLATE PUDDING

SERVES 6

This pudding can also be used as a pie filling. Consider using my Fresh Uncooked Piecrust (page 120). Of course, the pudding is also just great as it is. If you don't like nuts, simply leave them out.

    3 tablespoons arrowroot powder

    3 cups light coconut milk

    ½ cup agave nectar

    ¼ cup cocoa powder (NOW certified organic cocoa powder is great)

    ¼ teaspoon salt

    3 tablespoons walnuts (optional)

    1 teaspoon vanilla extract (sometimes I add a bit more, for extra vanilla flavor, but start with this)

- Place the arrowroot powder in a small bowl along with ½ cup of the coconut milk and whisk together really well until fully blended.
- In a saucepan, stir together the rest of the coconut milk with the agave nectar and cocoa powder, until well mixed. Heat this mixture to boiling, stirring with a whisk to dissolve the cocoa and blend everything together. This takes some whisking, as the cocoa powder doesn't dissolve quickly; be patient, the pudding is well worth the effort. As soon as the mixture comes to a boil, quickly stir in the arrowroot mixture and whisk. When the mixture begins to thicken, which won't take long, about a minute, turn off the heat and add the walnuts and vanilla. Stir well and pour into ramekins or individual bowls. Refrigerate until well chilled.

COCONUT RICE PUDDING

SERVES 4

I am a huge fan of rice pudding and sometimes I eat this for breakfast. I just add some chopped nuts and dates, and I am good to go! Try it. If you don't have cardamom pods, just add some cardamom powder or a pinch of nutmeg in place of the cardamom. It's so rich and creamy with the coconut milk!

1 cup uncooked brown rice

1 (14-ounce) can coconut milk

14 ounces (measure using above can) water

15 cardamom pods

¼ cup agave nectar

¼–½ teaspoon ground cinnamon

Pinch of sea salt

■ Rinse the rice in a colander and place in a saucepan with the coconut milk, water, and cardamom pods. Bring to boil, then lower the heat to low. Simmer over low heat until the pudding is thick and the rice is cooked through, about 45 minutes. Turn off the heat and add the agave nectar, cinnamon, and salt. Remove the cardamom pods and serve.

CRISPY RICE TREATS, HEALTHY STYLE

These are different *from the rice treats sold commercially. Because they are not loaded with sugar, they will wow your kids without sending them around the room like a spinning top. You can use other nut butters if you prefer, but the secret is really the puffed rice. It works great in this recipe. You can use other nuts and seeds if you wish. You can make these into squares or balls, whichever you prefer. I like the squares, so that is what I will describe here.*

2 cups puffed rice
¼ cup sesame seeds
¼ cup raw, chopped almonds
½ cup currants or raisins
¼ teaspoon ground cinnamon
¼ cup vegan chocolate chips
¼ teaspoon vanilla extract
¾ cup macadamia or cashew butter (or other nut butter of your choice)
¾ cup brown rice syrup

- Place the puffed rice, seeds, nuts, currants, cinnamon, and chocolate chips into a large bowl and mix together. In a smaller bowl, stir together the vanilla, brown rice syrup, and macadamia butter, then add this mixture to the puffed rice mixture. You need to stir this together really well so it will hold when cut into bars.
- Lightly spray a 9-inch square pan with vegetable oil nonstick spray and spoon the ingredients into the pan. With wet hands, spread the mixture out so it fills the pan. Refrigerate until well chilled, then cut into bars.

DELICIOUS BAKED APPLES

This recipe was a huge hit among my taste testers. They are especially good topped with Cashew Crème Frosting (page 171). I think part of the secret to their success is the basting process. If you baste these, while they are baking, with their own juices, they are delightful.

6 large Gala or other good baking apples, carefully cored but otherwise intact

¼ cup chopped walnuts

½ cup currants or raisins

¼–½ cup organic brown sugar (depending on how sweet the apples are)

1 teaspoon ground cinnamon

½ teaspoon grated nutmeg

6 tablespoons organic maple syrup

Cashew Crème Frosting (optional)

- Preheat the oven to 350°F.
- Set the apples in a square baking dish. In a small bowl, mix together the chopped walnuts, currants, organic brown sugar, cinnamon, and nutmeg. Carefully spoon this mixture into each apple, stuffing it down carefully so the apple is packed. Pour 1 tablespoon of the maple syrup over the top of each apple, then add about ½ cup of water to the bottom of the baking dish. Use the liquid from the apples mixed with water to marinate the apples while they are baking. (I do this two or three times during the baking process, and then again after they come out of the oven.) Bake until the apples are tender, 30–35 minutes. Be careful not to overcook them to the point that they fall apart!
- Serve these with a dollop of the Cashew Crème Frosting.

FROZEN BANANAS

This is a *good recipe for your young children to make. It doesn't make much of a mess, and they can get in there and push the nuts into the bananas. It's really quite fun. This is a very simple dessert that kids love!*

¼ cup finely ground walnuts or pecans (see Note)

2 large bananas, peeled

vegan semisweet chocolate chips (optional)

- Spread the nuts on a cutting board or counter, and carefully roll the banana in them, pressing the nuts into the fruit. Roll up the bananas into a piece of waxed paper and place it in the freezer. Freeze for at least an hour. You can also melt chocolate in a double boiler and then roll the bananas in the chocolate, then the nuts, and then wrap with the waxed paper.
- Unwrap and enjoy.

> Note: To achieve the best result, use a food processor to grind the nuts. If you don't have a food processor, you can substitute a blender, or just chop the nuts very fine.

GINGER RICE PUDDING

Ginger is so good for our digestion. It also has a very nice flavor, so I added it to this recipe and it was a hit. I think the combination of the coconut milk and the ginger really works well.

2 cups light coconut milk

½ cup water

1 cup uncooked Arborio rice

Pinch of sea salt

1 tablespoon finely chopped candied or fresh ginger

2–3 small Medjool dates, pitted and chopped

½ teaspoon ground cinnamon

■ Place the coconut milk and water in a pot and bring to a boil. Add the rice and the salt, and bring back to a boil. Turn down the heat, add the ginger and dates, and simmer over low heat for 40 to 45 minutes, or until the rice is cooked but not dried out. Rice pudding should be very moist. Add the cinnamon and serve!

PEACH AND BLUEBERRY COBBLER

SERVES 6

This is a party pleaser. You can substitute other fruits for the ones I have included here. Try nectarines or apples.

3 cups pitted, sliced peaches

3 cups blueberries

2 tablespoons sorghum flour

2 tablespoons organic brown sugar

2 tablespoons arrowroot powder

1½ teaspoons ground cinnamon

¾ cup sorghum flour

1 cup brown rice flakes, quinoa flakes, or certified-vegan oats

Pinch of sea salt

¼ cup sesame seeds

¼ cup chopped walnuts or pecans

¼ cup vegan margarine

¼ cup agave nectar or organic brown sugar

- Preheat the oven to 350°F. Lightly spray an 8- or 9 inch square pan with vegetable oil non-stick spray.
- Place the peaches in a large bowl. Add the blueberries, 2 tablespoons sorghum flour, 2 tablespoons brown sugar, arrowroot, and 1 teaspoon of the cinnamon, and mix together well.
- Pour the peach mixture into the pan.
- In a smaller bowl, combine the rest of the sorghum flour, brown rice flakes, remaining ½ teaspoon of cinnamon, salt, sesame seeds, and walnuts. Cut in the margarine with a fork or pastry cutter. Add the agave nectar and mix together really well. Crumble this over the top of the peach mixture and bake until bubbly, 30 to 35 minutes.

PEANUT BUTTER CANDY

This is another uncooked candy that will knock your socks off. Well, I hope it really doesn't do that literally, but I bet you can't eat just one! They are addictive, so share!

½ cup organic peanut butter

⅛ cup pitted and chopped Medjool dates

¼ cup chopped pecans

¼ cup sesame seeds

¼ cup brown rice syrup

1 tablespoon arrowroot powder

⅛ teaspoon ground cardamom

- Line a small cookie sheet or platter with baking parchment.
- Place all of the ingredients in a large mixing bowl and stir together until mixed really well. Roll into balls and place each ball on the prepared cookie sheet. Chill until set.

PEANUT BUTTER COOKIES

MAKES ABOUT 3 DOZEN

I took these cookies around town, and my friend Dan had a comment I found quite amusing. He said the cookies were good but that they needed "more nuts." Well, I thought that was funny since they are made with peanut butter and even have walnuts in them, but I took his comment to heart. I didn't add any more nuts mind you, but I listened. If you like a nuttier cookie, add more nuts.

1 cup vegan margarine or shortening

1 cup agave nectar

1½ teaspoons Ener-G egg replacer whisked together with 2 tablespoons warm water

½ cup applesauce

¼ teaspoon vanilla extract

1 cup peanut butter

1½ cups sorghum flour

¼ cup arrowroot powder

½ cup potato starch

2 teaspoons baking powder

½ teaspoon baking soda

½ teaspoon sea salt

1½ teaspoons xanthan gum

¾ cup vegan chocolate chips (Enjoy Life Foods brand, or other chips)

¾ cup chopped walnuts or peanuts

■ Preheat the oven to 350°F. Line a cookie sheet with baking parchment or lightly spray with vegetable oil nonstick spray.

■ In a large mixing bowl, combine the margarine and agave nectar, and beat together until smooth and creamy, 2 to 3 minutes. Add the egg substitute mixture and the applesauce, and mix well. Add the vanilla and peanut butter, and beat well. This mixture will look curdled, but that's okay.

■ In a separate bowl, sift together the sorghum flour, arrowroot, potato starch, baking powder, baking soda, salt, and xanthan gum. Add the dry mixture to the wet mixture and beat together. When thoroughly blended, add the chocolate chips and nuts, and stir to mix well.

■ Drop by spoonfuls onto the prepared cookie sheet. Dip a fork in cold water and flatten each cookie.

■ Bake for 18 to 20 minutes, or until lightly browned. Cool on a wire rack.

PEAR TORTE

This is a dessert to live for. Are you planning a party or going to a special gathering, and you want to bring something that will be appreciated by all of your gluten-free vegan friends? Make this recipe. They won't be disappointed.

Crust

½ cup vegan margarine

⅓ cup agave nectar

¼ teaspoon vanilla extract

¾ cup sorghum flour

⅔ cup chopped walnuts

Filling

1 (8-ounce) tub Tofutti soy cream cheese

1 tablespoon Tofutti soy sour cream

1½ teaspoons Ener-G egg replacer whisked together with 2 tablespoons warm water

½ teaspoon vanilla extract

⅛ cup agave nectar

1 pound pears, sliced lengthwise into quarters and cored

Ground cinnamon, for sprinkling

- Preheat the oven to 350°F. Lightly grease a 9-inch square baking pan with vegetable oil.
- Prepare the crust: Beat the margarine with the agave nectar until it is creamy. Add the rest of the crust ingredients. Stir to blend together well. Spread in the prepared pan and bake for 15 to 18 minutes, or until set. Let cool while you make the filling.
- For the filling: In a large mixing bowl, beat all the filling ingredients together (except the pears and cinnamon) until well blended. Pour over the cooled crust. Arrange the sliced pears on top of the filling. Sprinkle generously with cinnamon.
- Bake at 350 degrees until set, 20 to 30 minutes. Cool on a wire rack.

QUINOA COFFEE CAKE

SERVES 6 TO 8

This really tastes just like a coffee cake should taste, yet without the eggs, butter, or white flour. Yippie! Send this to school in your child's lunch box. Take it on a picnic. You won't be sorry.

Cake

- ½ cup agave nectar
- ¼ cup vegan margarine or coconut oil
- 1½ teaspoons Ener-G egg replacer whisked thoroughly with 2 tablespoons warm water
- 1 teaspoon vanilla extract
- ½ cup Tofutti soy sour cream
- ¼ cup water
- ½ cup applesauce
- 1¼ cups quinoa flour
- ¼ cup brown rice flour
- ⅓ cup tapioca flour
- 2 teaspoons baking powder
- 1 teaspoon baking soda
- 1 teaspoon ground cinnamon
- ½ teaspoon sea salt

Topping

- ½ cup quinoa flour
- ¼ cup organic brown sugar
- ¾ cup chopped nuts (walnuts, pecans, almonds, cashews, or a combination)
- ¼ teaspoon ground cinnamon
- ¼ cup vegan margarine, almond butter, or cashew butter

■ Preheat oven to 350°F. Lightly spray a 9-inch square pan with vegetable oil nonstick spray.

■ Prepare the cake: Place the margarine and agave nectar in a mixing bowl and beat together until the mixture is well blended. Add the egg replacer mixture, vanilla extract, soy sour cream, water, and applesauce, and stir well. In another bowl, combine all of the dry ingredients, then stir into the wet ingredients. Beat until well combined. Spoon the batter into the prepared baking dish.

■ Prepare the topping: Place the quinoa flour, brown sugar, nuts, and cinnamon in a small bowl. Cut in the margarine, using either a pastry cutter or your hands (clean of course), until the mixture is mixed well. Spread the topping over the cake batter and bake until browned, 35 to 40 minutes. Be sure to test the cake with a sharp knife or toothpick at the 30- to 35-minute mark (oven temperatures vary slightly). It should come out clean. Cool on wire rack and enjoy!

RASPBERRY TOFU PUDDING

SERVES 4

This is absolutely my favorite recipe. It is worth making over and over and over again. However, those of you with soy allergies should avoid this one. Make the Chocolate Pudding (page 142) instead. This pudding may also be used as a pie filling. Try the Fresh Uncooked Piecrust (page 126).

12 ounces extra-firm silken tofu

2 cups raspberries (frozen or fresh)

6 tablespoons agave nectar

2 teaspoons vanilla extract

Fresh mint, to garnish

- Place all of ingredients into a blender and puree until completely smooth. This may take 2 to 3 minutes. Immediately pour into ramekins or individual bowls, and place in the refrigerator. Garnish with fresh mint, if desired.
- If you are using fresh berries, it may be runnier than if you use frozen berries, so you will need to add some additional berries to make sure the pudding thickens appropriately ($\frac{1}{2}$ cup or so).

SUPER-DUPER FUDGE

My grandma used to make the best fudge. This version is not like hers, but I hope you like it as much as I do. You can leave out the maple butter if you don't have any—just increase the agave nectar to one cup. I first made this with only one cup of almond butter and it was delicious but a bit sticky, so I have increased the amount to one and a half cups. If you prefer it chewier, simply decrease the nut butter to one cup. Also, you can use other nuts or seeds in place of the walnuts, and/or add raisins, currants, or dates.

½ cup maple butter

½ cup agave nectar

1½ cups almond, cashew, macadamia, peanut, or hazelnut butter

½ cup organic cocoa

1 cup chopped walnuts

1 teaspoon vanilla extract

- Grease a square 8 or 9-inch or pan with a vegetable oil nonstick spray.
- Heat the maple butter, agave nectar, and almond butter in a 2-quart saucepan. When it is hot, turn off the heat and quickly add the cocoa powder, walnuts, and vanilla. Beat this mixture together rapidly, before it begins to thicken. Quickly pour the mixture into the prepared pan and spread around evenly. Place in the refrigerator until hard, then cut into squares.

TROPICAL PUDDING OR PIE FILLING

You have to eat this up quickly, as the banana will turn brown on the second day. Either reduce the amount of banana that you use and increase the amount of dates, or just eat it the first day and don't worry about it. I actually have a friend, Stephanie, who has been a taste tester of mine for a long time, and she says the pie tastes just as good on the second day as it does on the first. Her secret to making it look just as good on the second day is to just swirl the top around a bit: the brown from the bananas disappears! This is so versatile, add other fruits in season, or use different nuts. Use your imagination, the results are up to you.

1 cup peeled and mashed banana
2 cups peeled and pitted mango
½ cup diced pineapple
½ cup pitted dates
1 cup raw cashews
½–1 cup blueberries
2 tablespoons ground flax meal
Juice of 1 lime
½ teaspoon ground cinnamon
¼ teaspoon ground cardamom
Fresh Uncooked Piecrust (page 126) or other nonbaked crust (optional)

■ Place all the ingredients in a food processor and process until the mixture is completely blended and smooth. You can either serve this as a pudding (pour into ramekins and refrigerate until chilled) or use to fill my uncooked piecrust.

BEVERAGES

ALMOND MILK

BLUEBERRY SMOOTHIE

FRESH VEGGIE JUICE

HOT CHOCOLATE WITH COCONUT MILK

PEACH AND ALMOND SMOOTHIE

PEACH AND RASPBERRY SMOOTHIE

PROTEIN SMOOTHIE

ROASTED CAROB AND BRAZIL NUT SHAKE

STRAWBERRY SMOOTHIE

ALMOND MILK

This is the best almond milk I have ever had and I make it fresh every morning. You can use the pulp that is left over to make your own almond cheese, if you are feeling creative.

1 cup almonds

4 cups purified water

¼ cup agave nectar (or less if you prefer less sweetness)

¼ teaspoon vanilla extract

- Soak the almonds overnight, or for at least 6 hours, in a large bowl in the 4 cups of water. Pour the mixture into a blender or food processor and blend on high for 2 to 3 minutes, or until the milk is completely blended.
- Pour the milk through cheesecloth (I set my wire colander over a bowl in the sink, then I cover the colander with the cheesecloth and pour the mixture through that). Once the milk has flowed through, press the nut pulp against the cheesecloth with your hands to express all the liquid into the bowl.
- Return the strained milk to the blender and add the agave nectar and vanilla. Blend well and serve.

> Note: This will stay fresh in the refrigerator up to a week if you keep it in an airtight container.

BLUEBERRY SMOOTHIE

Blueberries are full of antioxidants and have been one of my favorite berries since I was a child. I love to put them in smoothies, cobblers, or crisps and use them in salads. I think you will find this smoothie very filling and satisfying.

2 cups blueberries
1 cup soy, nut, or rice milk
½ cup extra-firm silken tofu
5–6 ice cubes
Pinch of cinnamon
½ small banana (optional)

■ Place all of the ingredients in a blender and blend until smooth. Serve for breakfast or a morning pick-me-up.

FRESH VEGGIE JUICE

SERVES 1 (ABOUT 16 OUNCES)

If you prefer a sweeter juice, add some fresh squeezed orange juice to the mixture, or a little more apple.

2 cups well washed, chopped spinach

1 large beet, cut into small dices, plus its greens, washed well and chopped

6 large carrots, cut into small dices

4 large celery stalks, ends trimmed, cut into small dices

3 large apples, cored and cut into small dices

1 large cucumber, peeled and sliced thinly

2 large pears, cored and sliced thinly

- To juice these ingredients, run the spinach and beet greens through first, in small amounts, followed by the beet, carrots, celery, apples, cucumber, and pears to help push the green leafy vegetables through.
- After you have juiced all of the produce, stir the juice together and serve over ice, if you prefer it cold.

HOT CHOCOLATE
WITH COCONUT MILK

SERVES 4

Bruce wanted me to make a recipe for cocoa or hot chocolate. He said, "Come on, Suzi, I'll give you some coconut milk if you will develop some hot chocolate." So, here it is. It's a blend of two milks and some very good organic cocoa powder. No marshmallows, but who needs them?

1 cup light coconut milk
2 cup hemp or soy milk
¼ cup agave nectar
¼ cup organic cocoa powder

■ Heat the coconut and hemp milks in a 2-quart saucepan until it comes to a boil. Add the cocoa powder. Using a whisk, stir well. It's important to really whisk this together so the cocoa powder fully dissolves. Add the agave nectar and lower the heat to a simmer. Simmer for 5 minutes, or until the cocoa powder is completely dissolved and the mixture is heated through. Serve hot.

PEACH AND ALMOND SMOOTHIE

If you don't *have Medjool dates, use whatever kind you have, or substitute raisins or currants. They are added to provide fiber, so if you don't have any and feel you don't need the extra fiber, leave them out. It's up to you.*

4 large Medjool dates, pitted and chopped

2 cups hemp, soy, or almond milk

2 tablespoons agave nectar

¼ teaspoon vanilla extract

8–10 almonds, chopped

3 cups pitted, chopped peaches, fresh if possible

1–2 cups ice cubes (depending on how thick you like it)

¼ teaspoon nutmeg (optional)

■ Place all ingredients in a blender or food processor and blend on high until smooth, 2 to 3 minutes.

PEACH AND RASPBERRY SMOOTHIE

Peaches and raspberries *go so well together. I can't get enough of either of them in the summer. So, in the summer, please go to your local organic market and buy fresh produce, and in the winter, use frozen rather than canned fruit, as it isn't full of sugar.*

1½ cups pitted, chopped peaches (drained frozen peaches are OK, but fresh is better!)

1 cup raspberries

1 cup ice cubes

8–10 almonds

1 tablespoon agave nectar

2 dates, pitted and chopped

¼ teaspoon vanilla extract

1 cup soy, hemp, or almond milk

Fresh mint sprigs, for garnish (optional)

■ Put all ingredients, except the mint, in a blender and blend until smooth. Pour into glasses and serve with fresh mint, if desired.

PROTEIN SMOOTHIE

I often make this when I am on the run. It's quick, easy, and gives me that get-up-and-go that I need most at the beginning of the day. I like to use the Now brand of protein powder, in apple flavor. It's very good. Chocolate is also good, and a great combination with the bananas. If you don't have any protein powder, you can add more nuts or some tofu, or just leave the powder out; the smoothie will taste great with or without it.

- 1 scoop (about 1 tablespoon) protein powder (optional)
- 5–6 raw almonds
- 2 Medjool dates, pitted
- 2 fresh or dried figs, stemmed
- ½ banana, peeled
- 1 cup frozen or fresh raspberries
- ½ cup ice cubes
- 1 cup hemp, soy, or rice milk

■ Place all the ingredients in a blender and puree until smooth, 1 to 2 minutes. Serve immediately.

ROASTED CAROB
AND BRAZIL NUT SHAKE

SERVES 2

My friends loved this recipe. If you don't like Brazil nuts, try cashews or macadamia nuts; either will work great.

1¼ cup vanilla almond milk, or rice, soy, or hazelnut milk

1 medium-size banana, ripe and mashed

¼ cup organic carob powder

¾ cup coarsely chopped Brazil nuts

¼ cup agave nectar

½ teaspoon vanilla extract

½ teaspoon ground cinnamon

5–6 ice cubes

■ Place all the ingredients in a blender and blend on high until well blended. Pour into glasses and serve.

STRAWBERRY SMOOTHIE

SERVES 2

For me, smoothies are a great way to get my day off on the right track or to give me a pick-me-up in the middle of the day. This one is very filling and I can have a meal in minutes!

1 cup almond, hemp, soy, or rice milk

4–5 ice cubes

1 small banana, peeled and cut in half

¼ teaspoon vanilla extract

1 tablespoon ground flax meal

2 small Medjool dates

1 cup fresh or frozen strawberries

■ Place all of the ingredients into a blender and blend on high until very smooth, 1 to 2 minutes. Pour into glasses and serve immediately.

SAUCES AND CONDIMENTS

ALMOND BUTTER

ALMOND CHEESE

APPLE BUTTER

BALSAMIC SALAD DRESSING

BERRY SAUCE

CASHEW CRÈME FROSTING

CASHEW GRAVY

CHUNKY APPLESAUCE

EGGLESS MAYONNAISE

HERBED DRESSING

MANGO MADNESS SAUCE

PEANUT SAUCE

PESTO

PIZZA SAUCE

RASPBERRY VINAIGRETTE

RAW AVOCADO MAYO

ALMOND BUTTER

I love almonds; they are full of the "good" fats that we all need, so I eat them often. This is a quick easy recipe for almond butter. It is delicious on gluten-free, vegan waffles, stuffed into celery, or slathered on sliced apples. I am sure you will find many ways to serve it.

1½ cups raw almonds

2 teaspoons grapeseed or canola oil

Salt (optional)

- Preheat the oven to 350°F. Place the almonds on a cookie sheet that has been drizzled with the oil. Stir the nuts around, so they are lightly coated with the oil, and spread them out evenly. Check on the nuts after about 5 minutes, stirring to roast evenly. The almonds should be lightly toasted in 10 to 15 minutes.
- If desired, add salt; allow to cool completely. Place the nuts in a food processor and blend until smooth. This will take a few minutes to achieve the consistency of almond butter. If it is too dry, add a little oil and continue to blend.
- Store in an airtight container in the refrigerator.

ALMOND CHEESE

This is a great way to use the pulp left over from the almond milk recipe. I make the almond milk so often I could fill my refrigerator with this cheese. This is a basic version, but you could add other herbs and spices if you wish to make different varieties of cheese.

2 cups almond pulp (after you make almond milk, this is what is left over)

2 tablespoons olive or canola oil

2 tablespoons lemon juice

1 tablespoon nutritional brewer's yeast

1 teaspoon chopped chives

½ teaspoon sea salt

½ teaspoon organic garlic salt

■ When I make the almond milk (page 158), I pour it through a piece of cheesecloth. I really squeeze it so all of the milk comes out, then I put the pulp into a bowl and add the rest of the almond cheese ingredients. Stir together well. Wrap the mixture in the cheesecloth so it is in the shape of a log, and set it aside to ferment: Place this mixture on a plate over a bowl of hot water. After 2 hours pass, remove it from the plate and place it on a wire rack that is laid across another bowl. Then place a heavy pan or weight on top of the cheesecloth so that the weight pushes the remaining liquid from the almond cheese. Leave this over night. Then remove the weight and the cheesecloth, and form the cheese into a rectangle. Transfer to an airtight container and refrigerate. This can be used like cheese in many recipes. It will last for about 1 week if kept refrigerated.

APPLE BUTTER

This is absolutely delicious made with homemade applesauce (page 173) but, if you don't have time to make your own, don't sweat it. It smells so wonderful while it is cooking. Your whole house will smell like apples and cinnamon.

  1 (24-ounce) jar applesauce, or
    3 cups homemade
  2 cups organic brown sugar
  ½ teaspoon ground cinnamon
  ½ teaspoon freshly grated
    nutmeg
  ¼ cup white vinegar

■ Preheat the oven to 350°F. Mix all of these ingredients together well in a bowl and pour into a baking dish. Bake, uncovered, for about 2 hours, until the mixture is very thick. I stir this several times during the baking process. Once it cools, you can pour it into jars to give as gifts, or store in your refrigerator.

BALSAMIC SALAD DRESSING

This is a traditional dressing, not too fancy, not too plain. It's perfect for a salad any day. If you have fresh berries around, blend them in, or add some fresh rosemary out of the garden (not too much, just a pinch will do).

  3 tablespoons organic balsamic
    vinegar
  ½–¾ cup organic extra-virgin
    olive oil
  1 clove garlic, minced finely
  ¼ teaspoon salt
  Freshly ground pepper
  ½–1 teaspoon organic mustard

■ Place all of the ingredients in a blender or food processor, and process until well blended. Keep in the refrigerator.

BERRY SAUCE

I really like this sauce over my Blueberry Buckwheat Pancakes (page 110). It is can be poured over hot cereal, soy ice cream, or soy yogurt. I am sure you will find many other uses for it. You can substitute or add other berries in season, too.

1 cup raspberries

1 cup strawberries, hulled

⅛ cup water

¼ cup agave nectar

2 tablespoons arrowroot powder

¼ teaspoon ground cinnamon

■ Place the berries, water, and agave nectar in a saucepan and bring to a boil. Add the arrowroot and, using a whisk, stir briskly to help the arrowroot to dissolve. Bring back to a boil, then lower the heat. The mixture will begin to thicken. Keep stirring, and if the mixture gets too thick, thin it down with a little more water. Once the starch has cooked and the berries are soft, 5 to 8 minutes, add the cinnamon and remove from the heat.

CASHEW CRÈME FROSTING

This is a quick, easy, and healthier version of "frosting." I use it to top baked apples, and as a frosting for carrot cake (page 140) or gingerbread (page 127), and I am sure you will come up with your own ideas on how to serve it.

⅔ cup coconut milk

⅓ cup Medjool dates, pitted and chopped

1 cup raw cashews

½ teaspoon vanilla extract

■ Place all of the ingredients in a food processor or blender, and blend together until the consistency is very smooth. If it is too thick, add a touch more coconut milk to thin it slightly. If you can't find Medjool dates, use ordinary dates, but these have the best flavor and texture. Store in the refrigerator.

CASHEW GRAVY

This is wonderful served with No-Meat Meatballs (page 96), Nancy's Favorite Mushroom Nut Loaf (page 95), and even over pasta. Season to taste, and enjoy. Let your imagination run wild with this, using other herbs or spices, or finding new ways to serve it.

1¼ cups raw cashews

2 teaspoons wheat-free tamari sauce

1 teaspoon dried parsley

Pinch of Italian seasoning

1 teaspoon arrowroot powder

1 cup water

Sea salt

Freshly cracked pepper

- Preheat the oven to 300°F. Roast the cashews on a cookie sheet for about 15 minutes, or until very lightly browned.
- Place the cashews in a food processor and blend until very fine, almost flour- or pastelike. Add the tamari sauce, parsley, Italian seasoning, arrowroot powder, and water, and blend until smooth, 1 to 2 minutes.
- Pour the mixture into a 2-quart saucepan and heat to boiling, stirring constantly. You may need to add a bit more water to keep the mixture from becoming too thick, but I actually like it thick myself. Lower the heat and cook until heated through, about 1 to 2 minutes. If too thick, add a bit of water. Season to taste with the salt and pepper.

CHUNKY APPLESAUCE

There's nothing like homemade applesauce. My grandmother and my mom made homemade applesauce every summer when I was growing up. I made it for my kids, too. This is a new version of an older one, without all the sugar! There are many recipes in this book that call for applesauce. Here's a great recipe to use instead of store-bought versions. You can also add strawberries or blueberries to this mixture. You may also sweeten it with maple syrup instead of agave nectar. Be creative and enjoy.

6 large apples (such as organic Gala or Granny Smith)
Juice of 1 lemon or lime
¼ cup water
¼–½ cup agave nectar
½ teaspoon ground cinnamon

■ Place the apples, lemon juice, and water in a 2-quart saucepan and heat over medium-high heat. Once the water begins to boil, lower the heat and cover the saucepan. Steam-cook the apples until soft, stirring often to keep them from browning on top. When the apples begin to break down, add the agave nectar and cinnamon. Heat through and serve. The process takes 55 to 60 minutes for the applesauce to slowly cook and the flavors to blend.

EGGLESS MAYONNAISE

MAKES ABOUT 1 CUP

This is a quick and easy vegan version of traditional mayonnaise. Simple to make.

- ¾ cup organic extra-virgin olive oil
- ¼ cup sesame tahini
- ½ teaspoon mustard powder
- ¼ teaspoon sea salt
- 1–2 tablespoons lemon juice, freshly squeezed if possible
- ⅛ teaspoon freshly ground black pepper

- ■ Place all of the ingredients into a blender or food processor, and puree until smooth. Add more lemon juice to taste and adjust seasonings, depending on if you like your mayo mild or spicy. Store in an airtight container in the refrigerator for up to 2 weeks.

HERBED DRESSING

MAKES ABOUT ½ CUP

If you are on an "elimination diet" or want a dressing without any vinegar or too much spice, this dressing is for you. It is simple, yet delicious.

- 1 small shallot, minced finely
- 3 tablespoons lemon juice, freshly squeezed if possible
- ¼–⅓ cup organic olive oil
- 1 cup chopped fresh parsley
- 1 clove garlic, minced
- ¼ teaspoon sea salt
- Freshly ground pepper
- Fresh thyme or rosemary (optional)

- ■ Place all of the ingredients in a blender or food processor, and whip together until well blended. Store in an airtight container in the refrigerator.

MANGO MADNESS SAUCE

MAKES ABOUT 2 CUPS

This recipe is absolutely wonderful served over baked apples, or as a topping for my Coconut Pancakes (page 114) or Blueberry Buckwheat Pancakes (page 110). You can also use it over rice pudding (pages 144 and 147) or gingerbread (page 127)

2 teaspoons coconut oil or
    vegan margarine

2 cups chopped mangoes
    (frozen or fresh)

¾ cup agave nectar

1 tablespoon orange juice

¼ teaspoon ground cardamom

2 tablespoons arrowroot powder
    (adjust as needed)

1 teaspoon vanilla extract

Freshly cracked pepper (optional)

■ In a 2-quart saucepan, heat the coconut oil over medium heat and add the mangoes. Cook until the mangoes soften, about 5 minutes. Add the agave nectar, orange juice, cardamom, arrowroot, and vanilla, and continue to cook for another 5 to 6 minutes, or until the mixture begins to thicken. If your mangoes are juicy, you may need to adjust the amount of arrowroot, adding a bit more so the sauce will thicken. Season with cracked pepper, if desired.

PEANUT SAUCE

MAKES ABOUT 2 CUPS

This is a great sauce to serve with spring rolls (page 101). It is also very good served over rice noodles. Makes another quick and easy meal to serve up in a jiffy.

1¼ cups light coconut milk
⅓–½ cup organic peanut butter
2 tablespoons agave nectar
2 tablespoons wheat-free tamari sauce
¼–½ teaspoon red curry paste
Pinch of red pepper flakes
Pinch of sea salt (optional)

- Place all of the ingredients in a blender or food processor, and process until well blended.

PESTO

MAKES ABOUT ½ CUP

What I love about this recipe is the time it takes to make it: next to nothing. This is a quick, easy pesto that makes a meal in minutes. Boil some water, throw some noodles in a pot to cook, and you have dinner. I add pine nuts for protein. Serve with a salad and you are ready to eat!

¼–⅓ cup olive oil
1 cup chopped fresh basil
¼ cup chopped fresh parsley
2 tablespoons lemon juice
2–3 cloves garlic, minced
¼ teaspoon sea salt
Freshly cracked pepper
¼ cup pine nuts (optional)

- Place all of the ingredients in a blender or food processor, and process until well blended. I always put in the olive oil first, so it's at the bottom of the blender; this helps to blend the ingredients together. If it is too thick, add a little water to thin it so you can remove it easily from the blender or processer.

PIZZA SAUCE

This is my standard pizza sauce. *Sometimes I use pesto (page 176) for the base of my pizza, but when I want a tomato base, this is it!*

2 cloves garlic, chopped very finely

1 (6-ounce) can organic tomato paste

½ cup water

½ teaspoon salt

¼ teaspoon freshly ground pepper

1 teaspoon dried oregano

1 teaspoon dried basil

■ Place the garlic in a medium-size bowl. Add the tomato paste, water, salt, pepper, oregano, and basil. Stir to blend this mixture really well. Let it sit for 30 minutes so the flavors can blend together. Spread this mixture over your pizza crust (page 130) and add your favorite toppings.

RASPBERRY VINAIGRETTE

This recipe is great on Super Antioxidant Salad (page 51), but it can be used on mixed green salads, too.

1 cup raspberries (fresh or frozen)

⅛ cup balsamic or rice wine vinegar

⅓ cup organic extra-virgin olive oil

2 tablespoons agave nectar

¼ teaspoon salt

■ Whisk together all of the ingredients until well blended. Place in an airtight container and store in the refrigerator. This will last for up to a week in the fridge.

RAW AVOCADO MAYO

This is good on sandwiches, in lettuce wraps, or as a garnish on veggie burgers.

1 large avocado, peeled, pitted, and sliced

1 tablespoon fresh lime juice

½ cup pine nuts

1 clove garlic, minced

2 tablespoons organic apple cider vinegar (preferably Bragg's)

4–5 Medjool dates, pitted and cut in half

½–1 teaspoon sea salt

Pinch of cayenne

- Place all of the ingredients in a food processor or blender, and process on high until very smooth. If the mixture is too thick, thin it out a bit by adding a small amount of water so the consistency is smooth but not runny.

RESOURCES

WHERE CAN YOU FIND COMMON INGREDIENTS USED IN THIS BOOK?

SORGHUM FLOUR—I love this flour! I use it all the time. You can get it at health food stores, big chains, like Trader Joe's, Whole Foods Market, Wild Oats, Fresh Fields, PCC, Central Market, Marlene's Deli, Metropolitan Market, Fred Meyer, Safeway, and many other markets across the country.

AGAVE CACTUS NECTAR—This can be purchased at all the same places as above. You can also buy it wholesale from Whole Foods Market, in Gig Harbor, WA (253-851-8120, 888-835-2312), and Enjoy Life Foods, in Chicago, IL (773-889-5070). If you order from either of these places, be sure to tell them Suzi O'Brien sent you.

ARROWROOT POWDER—This is used to thicken sauces, or added to baked goods in place of cornstarch. Since I use it so often, I recommend you buy it and keep it in the pantry. It is available at all the places mentioned in the sorghum flour recommendations above.

BROWN RICE FLOUR—Again, found at all the places mentioned above, along with your regular grocery stores. Just look in one of two places, the health food section of the store, or the flour section. It is becoming very common to find this flour in all grocery stores (with the exception of your small mom and pop stores).

XANTHAN GUM—This is used to thicken liquids, or to help baked goods stay together. What happens when you remove gluten from baked goods is that they tend to become crumbly, and fall apart easily. Xanthan gum helps to bind the ingredients together. This can be found at health food stores, some local grocery stores, and, of course, on line, or at any major health food chain, such as Whole Foods Market.

ORGANIC SHORTENING—I use Spectrum, because it is non-GMO, trans-fat free, dairy-free, and gluten-free. It really is great in piecrusts. You can find it in any health food store, and most of the places mentioned above. Even our Safeway carries it, Ralph's in California, and Fred Meyer. Or look in the freezer case of health food stores and large supermarkets for Earth Balance Buttery Spread or Shortening, which are both 100 percent vegan and gluten free, and come in sticks like butter.

SOY MILK—I use soy milk in many things. If you have a soy allergy, think about the consistency of the recipe, then consider your options. If you are making gravy, rice or almond milk will be fine in place of soy, but if you are adding the milk to a curry stir-fry, rice milk won't do. You may want to consider adding some coconut milk in place of soy. Before making any substitution for soy milk in my recipes, think about how flavor and consistency will be affected.

QUINOA—This is a wonderful grain. This can be found in all places mentioned above, as well as your everyday grocery store. Look in the grain section, if you are at your supermarket; it will be prepackaged. If you are at the health food store, you can buy it in bulk, or prepackaged. It's great to have in the pantry, as you can toss it in soups, salads, and so on, and it adds a wonderful nutty flavor as well as protein and fiber.

POTATO STARCH AND TAPIOCA STARCH—These ingredients can be found in all the places mentioned above and are used frequently in my recipes as wheat flour replacements.

FRUITS, VEGETABLES, BERRIES, NUTS, SEEDS, AND GRAINS—These ingredients are so important to have in the house. You can cook anything if you have the basics in the freezer, fridge, pantry, and fruit bowl. Keep these around so you make healthy choices regarding your meals and snacks. You'll feel better, and in the long term, you will stay healthy longer as you age. Be sure to buy locally and get the freshest fruits and veggies you can find. If you have a food co-op nearby, consider joining, or check around to see if your local farms sell and deliver organic produce. Many are doing that now, and you can sign up for weekly deliveries from spring until late fall.

RESOURCE GUIDE FOR GLUTEN-FREE, VEGAN PRODUCTS

MY LOCAL HEALTH food store (Whole Foods Market, in Gig Harbor) is wonderful because they will order any product that I need that is not on the shelf. If you cannot find my recipes' ingredients at your local grocery store, find a health food store or a gourmet food/supermarket that carries organic foods, as they will probably have them. Wild Oats, Whole Foods Markets, and Fresh Fields grocery stores all carry a wealth of gluten-free, dairy-free, sugar-free products. If they don't, ask them to order for you. If you don't have a health food store nearby, consider ordering supplies via the Internet. I have listed some resources here for you.

Allergy Resources
PO Box 444
Guffy, CO 80820
They will send you a free catalog.

Arrowhead Mills, Inc.
PO Box 2059
Hereford, TX 79045
800-364-0730
Wheat-free grains, beans, oils, flours, mixes, ready-to-eat cereals, butters.

Bob's Red Mill Natural Foods
5209 S.E. International Way
Milwaukee, OR 97222
503-654-3215
Wheat-free flours, pastas, baking mixes, soup mixes, xanthan and guar gum, etc.

Brumwell Flour Mill
328 East Second Street, Box 233
Sumner, IA 50674
319-578-8106
Organic flours, including oat, corn, and buckwheat. They will also grind unroasted buckwheat if requested.

Celiac.com
(www.celiac.com) is a wonderful Web site for everything you need to know about avoiding gluten in the diet. They have lists of "forbidden" foods, links to other resources, and a wonderful bookstore, too. If you are allergic to gluten, or need to avoid all products containing gluten, I highly recommend this site. It will provide you with a wealth of information.

Dixie Diner
www.dixiediner.com
Offers a link to lots of gluten-free vegan foods you can purchase online.

Ener-G Foods, Inc.
PO Box 84487
Seattle, WA 98124
800-331-5222
Gluten-free flours, egg replacer, lacto-free foods.

Enjoy Life Foods
1601 N. Natchez
Chicago, IL 60707
1-888-50-enjoy or 773-889-5070
www.enjoylifefoods.com
Many wonderful products, all dairy-free, egg-free, soy-free, gluten-free, GMO-free, and kosher. They also will ship bulk agave nectar. Ask for Bert! Tell him Sue sent you.

Earth Balance
GFA Brands, Inc.
PO Box 397
Cresskill, NJ 07626-0397
201-568-9300
www.earthbalance.net
Specializing in nonhydrogenated, 100 percent vegan margarine and shortening and tub-style whipped spreads that are both gluten-free and dairy-free.

Follow Your Heart Vegan Gourmet
Box 9400
Canoga Park, CA 91309-0400
818-348-3240
e-mail: marick@followyourheart.com
Many dairy- and gluten-free cheeses, in several flavors.

Galaxy Foods
2441 Viscount Row
Orlando, FL 32809
1-800-808-2325
www.galaxyfoods.com
Specializes in many gluten-free, dairy-free cheeses. Carries a sour cream substitute, as well as many different flavors and textures of cheese alternatives.

Lundberg Family Farms
PO Box 369
Richvale, CA 95974
916-882-4551
www.lundberg.com
They carry brown rice, Wehani rice, and rice medleys, brown rice syrup, rice cakes, and cereals.

Mrs. Leeper's Pasta
12455 Kerran Street #200
Poway, CA 92064
This is my all-time favorite for wheat-free pasta! They carry corn and rice flour pasta, and sauces, too.

Organic Wine Company
www.ecowine.com
Offers six varieties of organic, vegan wines.

Road's End Organics
120 Pleasant Street, E-1
Morrisville, VT 05661
1-877-247-3373
www.chreese.com
They carry a nondairy cheese that is made from lentil flour. They also carry various flavors of cheese and dips.

Spectrum Natural Organic Products, Inc.
5341 Old Redwood Highway, Suite 400
Petaluma, CA 94954
www.spectrumnaturals.com
Many wonderful organic products, including vegan shortening that is nonhydrogenated and trans fat–free.

Sweet Cactus Farms
10627 Regent Street
Los Angeles, CA 90034
310-733-4343
e-mail: agave@sweetcactusfarms.com
Agave cactus nectar is a vegan, gluten-free sugar alternative. It is very low on the glycemic index and is a great substitute for sugar.

Thermosweet
Customer service: 100 2nd Avenue South
200 South Tower
St. Petersburg, FL 33701
e-mail: nutrilabcorp@aol.com
Manufactures kiwi sweeteners.

Twin Valley Mills
RR 1, Box 45
Ruskin, NE 68974
402-279-3965
www.twinvalleymills.com
Sorghum flour in bulk.

Vegan Connection
www.veganconnection.com
Offers many links to helpful resources.

Vitasoy, USA, Inc.
One New England Way
Ayer, MA 01432
1-800-vitasoy
Aside from soy milks, their Nasoya division makes a dairy-free, egg-free mayonnaise. It is called Nayonaise, and it is great!

Whole Foods Market
PO Box 244
Gig Harbor, WA 98335
1-888-835-2312
A good source for many products, especially for wholesale agave nectar (1 gallon size). Ask for Bruce, and tell him Suzi sent you.

ACKNOWLEDGMENTS

T HERE ARE MANY people to thank for their generous gifts of support and assistance with this book. I want to begin with my family at the Whole Foods Market in Gig Harbor, Washington. Bruce Winfrey and Nancy Moffitt were incredible taste testers and an invaluable source of support during the development of this book. I thank you both very much for your loving kindness and honest opinions.

There were taste testers from every walk of life involved in this book, those who have no interest in health foods or veganism, and those who have a vested interest in eating a healthy, gluten-, dairy-, and egg-free diet. There were those who indeed are vegans, and others who live with food allergies. Even strangers, who happened to be at the Whole Foods Market when I was dropping off samples, offered to be taste testers. Not only did everyone agree that the recipes were great, but those who never ate gluten-free, vegan food said they would choose to make these recipes for their families because they were so chock-full of taste and texture. My sincere thanks to all of you.

I also want to thank Dara Morgan for her hard work typing my recipes from scraps of paper ranging from torn-off envelopes to three recipes written on a tablet sideways! Not only did she help type the recipes so you could all enjoy them, she tested them as she typed. You rock, Dara! Kathy Cseke, thank you so much for your excellent editing skills. I appreciate you taking the time to read the opening sections as well as the recipes and for providing excellent suggestions and improvements. I am very grateful to Katie McHugh at Marlowe and Company for all of her editing work and patience with my very hectic schedule. Thank you, Barb, for writing the introduction to this book. You have been a guiding light for me, and I am grateful for your contributions to all of my cookbooks. Special thanks to Lewis Perkin for permissions to use his Yam Enchiladas with Pomegranate recipe.

To Carol Dudley, my best friend, you have always been the calm in the storm for me, the person who reminds me that in breathing in, I am. I live in gratitude for our friendship.

I also want to acknowledge my mom for gifting me with her passion, her creative energy, and her love of life.

I would like to thank the following people for being my taste testers: Cary Perkins, Barb Schiltz, Sally Priest, Sheila Quinn, Dara Morgan, Marcia Doran, James Traub, Zack Rosenbloom, Liz Merrit, Debbie Freisen, Maggie Hagler, Jim O'Brien, Terry O'Brien, Jeffrey Fors, Jessie Bjorklund, Rory O'Brien-Berthiaume, Sam Burkhart, Mike and Steve Burkhart, Stephanie Ann, Anna Columbini, ND, the staff at the Peninsula Naturopathic Clinic in Gig Harbor, Paul Reilly, ND, and his staff, the entire staff at the Functional Medicine Research Center in Gig Harbor, Daniel and Holly Roso, Chris Holts, Jen, Skylar, Zane, and Brad Lantz, Brent Holbrook, and Dan Lukaczer, who advised me to add more nuts to the peanut butter cookies!

I would also like to acknowledge those who provided tremendous encouragement and support along the way, including my sons, Jeff and Rory, who are a constant source of love and joy, my dad and brothers, Jessie Bjorklund, Connie Harrington, Kathy Granger, Pat Bujacich, Karen McDonnell, and my dear friend Stephanie Ann.

Thank you all with love and gratitude,

SUSAN

INDEX

agave cactus nectar, 7, 179
Allergy Resources, 181
almond
    almond butter, 168
    almond cheese, 169
    almond meal flour, 12
    almond milk, 9, 158
    peach and almond
        smoothie, 162
antioxidant chili, 84
antioxidant risotto, 85
antioxidant salad, 51
appetizers, 19–27
    apple salsa, 20
    black bean salsa, 21
    curried bean dip, 22
    guacamole, 23
    hummus, 24
    maple candied nuts, 25
    salsa, 26
    spicy mixed nuts and
        seeds, 27
apples
    apple butter, 170
    apple pie bars, 134
    apple-raspberry pie
        filling, 135
    apple salsa, 20
    chunky applesauce, 173
    curried apple and cauli-
        flower soup, 30
    delicious baked apples,
        141
applesauce, 173
Arrowhead Mills, 181

arrowroot, 13
    powder, 179
asparagus
    asparagus risotto, 86
    grilled asparagus, 60
autism spectrum conditions, 4
avocado
    fresh avocado and
        cucumber soup, 33
    guacamole, 23
    raw avocado mayo, 178

baking powder, 14, 120
baking soda, 14
balsamic salad dressing, 170
bananas, frozen, 146
bars
    apple pie bars, 134
    cranberry granola bars,
        123
bean dip, curried, 22
beans
    bean salad, 42
    black, 21, 57, 91
    black beans, 57
    black bean salsa, 21
    curried bean dip,
        22
    fava bean and vegetable
        soup, 32
    green, 59, 75
    green beans with
        edamame, 59
    salt and pepper
        edamame, 73

Slavonian-style green
        beans, 75
    soybeans, 59, 73
    tomato and white bean
        soup, 40
    white beans, 40
    yam and black bean
        burritos, 91
beets
    herbed beets and onion
        gratin, 61
    roasted beets, 69
bell peppers
    roasted red bell peppers,
        71
    veggie-stuffed bell
        peppers, 106
berry and cherry crisp, 137
berry sauce, 171
beverages, 157–166
    almond milk, 158
    blueberry smoothie,
        159
    hot chocolate with
        coconut milk, 161
    peach and almond
        smoothie, 162
    peach and raspberry
        smoothie, 163
    protein smoothie, 164
    roasted carob and Brazil
        nut shake, 165
    strawberry smoothie, 166
    vegetable juice, 160
biscuits, 120

black beans, 57
    black bean salsa, 21
    yam and black bean
        burritos, 91
blood glucose, 5
blood sugar, 5
blueberry
    blueberry buckwheat
        pancakes, 110
    blueberry smoothie,
        159
    peach and blueberry
        cobbler, 148
Bob's Red Mill Natural
    Foods, 10, 181
Brand-Miller, Jennie, 6
Brazil nut and roasted
    carob shake, 165
breads
    carrot bread, 121
    cornbread, 122
    gingerbread, 127
breakfast foods, 109–117
    blueberry buckwheat
        pancakes, 110
    breakfast rice with fruit,
        111
    breakfast risotto, 112
    breakfast vegetable bake,
        113
    coconut pancakes, 114
    granola, 115
    potato and tofu hash,
        116
    tofu scramble, 117
brownies, 138
brown rice, 15–16
    flour, 11, 179
    syrup, 6, 134
    tortillas, 10
Brumwell Flour Mill, 181
buckwheat flour, 11
    blueberry buckwheat
        pancakes, 110
burgers, veggie, 105
Burke, Cindy, 2
burritos, yam and black
    bean, 91
butter, 8
    almond butter,
        168
    apples butter,
        170
butternut squash

butternut squash dessert,
    139
    stuffed butternut squash,
        78

cabbage, and ginger sauté,
    58
cake
    carrot cake, 140
    quinoa coffee cake, 152
candy, peanut butter, 149
carbohydrate content, 5–6
carob
    roasted carob and Brazil
        nut shake, 165
carrots
    carrot bread, 121
    carrot cake, 140
    carrot salad, 43
casein-free diet, 3–4
cashews
    cashew crème frosting,
        171
    cashew gravy, 172
casserole, spring, 100
cauliflower, 30
    curried apple and cauli-
        flower soup, 30
celiac disease, 4–5, 128, 181
Central Market, 179
cheese, almond, 169
cherries
    berry and cherry crisp,
        137
chili
    antioxidant chili, 84
    tofu chili, 102
chocolate
    chocolate chip cookies,
        141
    chocolate pudding, 142
    hot chocolate with
        coconut milk, 161
    no-bake chocolate
        cookies, 136
cholesterol, 8
chowder, corn, 31
cobbler, peach and
    blueberry, 148
coconut
    coconut pancakes,
        114
    coconut rice pudding,
        143

curried coconut and
    squash stew, 87
    hot chocolate with
        coconut milk, 161
    milk, 9
    oil, 8
coffee cake, quinoa, 152
coleslaw, 54
condiments, 167–178
    almond butter, 168
    almond cheese, 169
    apple butter, 170
    balsamic salad dressing,
        170
    berry sauce, 171
    cashew crème frosting,
        171
    cashew gravy, 172
    chunky applesauce, 173
    eggless mayonnaise, 174
    herbed dressing, 174
    mango madness sauce,
        175
    peanut sauce, 176
    pesto, 176
    pizza sauce, 177
    raspberry vinaigrette,
        177
    raw avocado mayo,
        178
cookies
    chocolate chip, 141
    no-bake chocolate, 136
    peanut butter, 150
corn chowder, 31
cornbread, 122
cornmeal, 16
cornstarch, 13
cranberry granola bars, 123
crisps, berry and cherry, 137
crusts
    fresh uncooked piecrust,
        126
    piecrust, 129
    pizza crust, 130
cucumbers
    avocado and cucumber
        soup, 33
    cucumber salad, 44
currant scone, 124
curry
    curried apple and cauli-
        flower soup, 30
    curried bean dip, 22

curried coconut and
squash stew, 87
potato and pea curry, 68

dairy alternatives, 3–4
dates, 162
desserts, 133–155
apple pie bars, 134
apple-raspberry filling,
135
baked apples, 145
berry and cherry crisp,
137
brownies, 138
butternut squash dessert,
139
carrot cake, 140
chocolate chip cookies,
141
chocolate pudding,
142
coconut rice pudding,
143
crispy rice treats, 144
frozen bananas, 146
fudge, 154
ginger rice pudding,
147
no-bake chocolate
cookies, 136
peach and blueberry
cobbler, 148
peanut butter candy,
149
peanut butter cookies,
150
pear torte, 151
quinoa coffee cake, 152
raspberry tofu pudding,
153
tropical pudding or pie
filling, 155
dips
apple salsa, 20
black bean salsa, 21
curried bean dip, 22
guacamole, 23
hummus, 24
salsa, 26
Dixie Diner, 181
dosas, 125
dressing
balsamic salad dressing,
170

herbed dressing, 174
raspberry vinaigrette, 177

Earth Balance, 8, 180–181
edamame
green beans with
edamame, 59
salt and pepper
edamame, 73
eggplant roll-ups, 88
egg substitutes, 9–10
enchiladas, yam with pomegranate sauce, 107
Ener-G Foods, 9, 14, 181
Enjoy Life Foods, 179, 181

fava bean and vegetable
soup, 32
flour, 10–13
almond meal, 12
brown rice, 11, 179
buckwheat, 11
garbanzo bean, 11
lentil, 11
potato, 12
quinoa, 11
sorghum, 12, 179
soy, 12
tapioca, 12
white rice, 11
Follow Your Heart Vegan
Gourmet, 182
Fred Meyer, 179–180
French Meadow Bakery, 10
Fresh Fields, 10, 179, 181
fritters, vegetable, 80
frosting, cashew crème, 171
fruits
breakfast rice with fruit,
111
fruit and nut salad, 45
fudge, 154

Galaxy Foods, 182
garbanzo bean flour, 11
genetically engineered and
modified organisms
(GMO), 2–3
Gifts of Nature, 10
ginger
cabbage and ginger
sauté, 58
gingerbread, 127
ginger rice pudding, 147

gingerbread, 127
gluten-free diet, 4–5
foods to avoid, 13
gluten/wheat substitutes,
10–13
See also flour
glycemic index (GI), 5
GMO foods (genetically
engineered and modified
organisms), 2–3
Good Carb Cookbook: Secrets of
Eating Low on the Glycemic
Index (Woodruff), 6
grains, 15–16
brown rice, 15–16
cornmeal, 16
millet, 15
oats, 15
polenta, 16
quinoa, 15
wild rice, 16
granola, 115
cranberry granola bars, 123
grapeseed oil, 8
gravy, cashew, 172
green beans
green beans with
edamame, 59
Slavonian-style green
beans, 75
guacamole, 23

hash, potato and tofu, 116
Healthy Hemp, 10
hemp tortillas, 10
honey, 7
hummus, 24

internet, 6

juice, vegetable, 160

kale with peanut sauce, 62

lactose, 3–4
lauric acid, 9
leek sauté, 63
lentil flours, 11
lentils
lentil stew, 92
spinach dal, 76
lettuce wraps, 93
Greek-style, 93
Mexican-style, 93

Living Without magazine, 10–13
Lundberg Family Farms, 6, 182

main dishes, 83–107
    antioxidant chili, 84
    antioxidant risotto, 85
    asparagus risotto, 86
    curried coconut and
        squash stew, 87
    eggplant roll-ups, 88
    Italian risotto, 89
    Italian-style pasta, 90
    yam and black bean
        burritos, 91
    lentil stew, 92
    lettuce wraps, 93
    mushroom and olive
        pizza, 94
    mushroom nut loaf, 95
    no-meat meatballs, 96
    Pad Thai, 97
    spaghetti squash with
        vegetable ragout, 98
    spicy quinoa pilaf, 99
    spring casserole, 100
    spring rolls, 101
    tofu chili, 102
    vegetable paella, 103
    vegetable ratatouille over
        rice, 104
    veggie burgers, 105
    veggie-stuffed bell
        peppers, 106
    yam enchiladas with
        pomegranate sauce,
        107
mango sauce, 175
maple butter, 7
maple syrup, 7
margarine, 8
Marlene's Deli, 179
mayonnaise
    eggless mayonnaise, 174
    raw avocado mayo, 178
meatballs, no-meat, 96
Medjool dates, 162
Metropolitan Market, 179
milks, 8–9
    almond, 9, 158
    coconut, 9, 161
    rice, 9
    soy, 8–9, 180

millet, 13, 15
minestrone soup, 36
molasses, 7
monolaurian, 9
Mrs. Leeper's Pasta, 182
mushrooms
    mushroom and olive
        pizza, 94
    mushroom nut loaf, 95
    mushroom sauté, 65
    stuffed Portobello
        mushrooms, 79
Mystic Lake Dairy, 6

*New Glucose Revolution: The
Authoritative Guide to the
Glycemic Index* (Brand-Miller
    and Wolever), 6
nuts, 14
    fruit and nut salad, 45
    maple candied nuts, 25
    mushroom nut loaf, 95
    roasted carob and Brazil
        nut shake, 165
    spicy mixed nuts and seeds,
        27

oats, 5, 15
    oat scones, 128
oils, 8
olive oil, 8
olives, and mushroom pizza,
    94
onions, and herbed beets
    gratin, 61
organic foods, 1–2
organic shortening, 180
Organic Wine Company, 182

Pad Thai, 97
paella, vegetable, 103
palm shortening, 8
pancakes
    blueberry buckwheat,
        110
    coconut, 114
    dosas, 125
pasta, Italian-style, 90
PCC, 179
peaches
    peach and almond
        smoothie, 162
    peach and blueberry
        cobbler, 148

peach and raspberry
    smoothie, 163
peanut butter
    peanut butter candy,
        149
    peanut butter cookies,
        150
peanut sauce, 62, 77, 176
pears
    pear torte, 151
    spinach and pear salad,
        50
peas, and potato curry,
    68
peppers
    roasted red bell peppers,
        71
    veggie-stuffed bell
        peppers, 106
pesto, 176
piecrust, 126, 129
pie filling
    apple-raspberry, 135
    tropical pudding or pie
        filling, 155
pilaf, spicy quinoa, 99
pine nuts, with sautéed
    spinach, 74
pizza
    crust, 130
    mushroom and olive,
        94
    sauce, 177
polenta, 16, 67
pomegranate sauce, yam
    enchiladas with, 107
Portobello mushrooms,
    stuffed, 79
potato
    and pea curry, 68
    and tofu hash, 116
    flour, 12
    mashed sweet potatoes,
        64
    not-fried potatoes,
        66
    roasted with herbs,
        70
    starch, 12, 180
    sweet potato salad, 52
product guide, 181–182
pudding
    chocolate, 142
    coconut rice, 143

ginger rice, 147
raspberry tofu, 153
tropical, 155
pumpkin scones, 131

quinoa, 15, 180
and vegetable salad, 49
coffee cake, 152
flour, 11
Mexican quinoa salad, 47
spicy quinoa pilaf, 99

Ralph's, 180
raspberry
and apple pie filling, 135
and peach smoothie, 163
tofu pudding, 153
vinaigrette, 177
ratatouille, vegetable, 104
raw foods, 2–3
rice, 15–16
and vegetable soup, 37
breakfast rice with fruit,
111
brown, 15–16
coconut rice pudding,
143
crispy rice treats, 144
flour, 12
ginger rice pudding, 147
milk, 9
wild, 16
with vegetable ratatouille,
104
risotto
antioxidant, 85
asparagus, 86
breakfast, 112
Italian, 89
Road's End Organics, 182
roll-ups, eggplant, 88

Safeway, 179–180
salads, 41–54
bean, 42
carrot, 43
coleslaw, 54
cucumber, 44
fruit and nut, 45
garden, 46
Mexican quinoa, 47
mock tabbouleh, 48
quinoa and vegetable, 49
spinach and pear, 50

super antioxidant, 51
sweet potato, 52
Waldorf, 53
salsa, 26
apple, 20
black bean, 21
sauces
applesauce, 173
berry sauce, 171
mango, 175
peanut, 62, 77, 176
pizza, 177
pomegranate, 107
sauté
cabbage and ginger, 58
leek, 63
mushroom, 65
scones
currant, 124
oat, 128
pumpkin, 131
seeds, 14
and spiced mixed nuts, 27
Shady Maple Farms, 7
shake, roasted carob and
Brazil nut, 165
shortenings, 8
side dishes, 55–81
baked delicata squash, 56
black beans, 57
cabbage and ginger
sauté, 58
green beans with
edamame, 59
grilled asparagus, 60
herbed beets and onion
gratin, 61
kale with peanut sauce,
62
leek sauté, 63
mashed sweet potatoes,
64
mushroom sauté, 65
not-fried potatoes, 66
polenta, 67
potato and pea curry, 68
roasted beets, 69
roasted potatoes with
herbs, 70
roasted red bell peppers,
71
roasted vegetables, 72
salt and pepper
edamame, 73

sautéed spinach with pine
nuts, 74
Slavonian-style green
beans, 75
spinach dal, 76
spinach tofu with peanut
sauce, 77
stuffed butternut squash,
78
stuffed Portobello
mushrooms, 79
vegetable fritters, 80
vegetable stir-fry, 81
smoothies
blueberry, 159
peach and almond, 162
peach and raspberry, 163
protein, 164
sorghum flour, 12, 179
soups, 29–40
avocado and cucumber,
33
corn chowder, 31
curried apple and
cauliflower, 30
fava bean and vegetable,
32
homemade vegetable
stock, 34
Mediterranean, 35
minestrone, 36
rice and vegetable, 37
roasted tomato, 38
Thai vegetable, 39
tomato and white bean,
40
soybeans, 59, 73
soy flour, 12
soy milk, 8–9, 180
spaghetti squash with vegetable ragout, 98
Spectrum Natural Organic
Products, 8, 180, 182
spinach
and pear salad, 50
sautéed with pine nuts,
74
dal, 76
tofu with peanut sauce, 77
spring rolls, 101
squash
baked delicata, 56
butternut squash dessert,
139

curried coconut and
squash stew, 87
spaghetti squash with
vegetable ragout, 98
stuffed butternut squash,
78
starches, 180
stew
curried coconut and
squash, 87
lentil, 92
stock, vegetable, 34
strawberry smoothie,
166
sugar alternatives, 6–7
agave cactus nectar, 7
brown rice syrup, 6
maple butter, 7
maple syrup, 7
molasses, 7
Sweet Cactus Farms, 182
sweeteners, 6–7
sweet potato
mashed, 64
salad, 52

tabbouleh, 48
tapioca flour, 12
tapioca starch, 12, 180
Thai foods, 39, 97
Thermosweet, 182
To Buy or Not to Buy Organic
(Burke), 2
tofu
potato and tofu hash, 116
raspberry tofu pudding,
153
scramble, 117
spinach tofu with peanut
sauce, 77

tofu chili, 102
Tofutti, 3
tomato
and white bean soup, 40
roasted tomato soup, 38
torte, pear, 151
tortillas, 10
Trader Joe's, 10, 179
trans fats, 1
Twin Valley Mills, 182

vegan, 1
Vegan Connection, 182
vegetable dishes, 55–81
baked delicata squash, 56
black beans, 57
cabbage and ginger
sauté, 58
green beans with
edamame, 59
grilled asparagus, 60
herbed beets and onion
gratin, 61
kale with peanut sauce,
62
leek sauté, 63
mashed sweet potatoes,
64
mushroom sauté, 65
not-fried potatoes, 66
polenta, 67
potato and pea curry, 68
roasted beets, 69
roasted potatoes with
herbs, 70
roasted red bell peppers,
71
roasted vegetables, 72
salt and pepper
edamame, 73

sautéed spinach with pine
nuts, 74
Slavonian-style green
beans, 75
spinach dal, 76
spinach tofu with peanut
sauce, 77
stuffed butternut squash,
78
stuffed Portobello
mushrooms, 79
vegetable fritters, 80
vegetable stir-fry, 81
vinaigrette, raspberry, 177
Vitasoy, 182

Waldorf salad, 53
Wax Orchards, 6–7
Westbrae Foods, 182
wheat, 4
white bean, and tomato
soup, 40
white rice flour, 11
Whole Foods Market, 10,
179, 181–182
Wild Oats, 10, 179, 181
wild rice, 16
Wolever, Thomas M.S., 6
Woodruff, Sandra L., 6
wraps, lettuce, 93
Greek-style, 93
Mexican-style, 93

xanthan gum, 179–180

yam and black bean burritos,
91